Pattern Setting for Childhood Health

The Parent's Guide for Nutrition and Activity

By Susan Garson, R.N., SANE-A

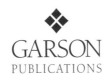

GARSON

PUBLICATIONS

Pattern Setting for Childhood Health

The Parent's Guide for Nutrition and Activity

by Susan Garson, R.N., SANE-A

Copyright ©2003 by Susan Garson
ISBN 0-9743496-0-7

Published by:

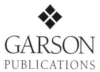

GARSON
PUBLICATIONS

Post Office Box 5775
Salem, Oregon 97304
☎ (503) 363-1477
FAX: (503) 363-1417
Website: www.susangarson.com
Printed in the United States of America

Table of Contents

About the Author

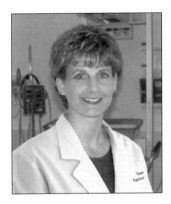

Susan Garson is a Registered Nurse with a primary focus in caring for hospitalized pediatric patients. As need dictates, she also works on other units such as maternal-child, special care nursery, medical, surgical, orthopedic, oncology, and psychiatry.

In addition to hospital floor nursing, Susan manages a specialized emergency room Sexual Assault Team. Under her direction, nurses help traumatized victims of all ages through the delicate process of acute medical and psychological treatment while performing an extensive and necessary forensic evidence collection examination. Susan is a sought-after lecturer, consultant, and writer on the subject.

As a volunteer member, Susan serves on the Marion County (Oregon) Child Abuse and Fatality Review Team and Multi-disciplinary Sexual Assault Team. She is also in the process of creating a specialized child abuse detection and prevention team in her hospital.

In order to help mothers with new babies make a smooth lifestyle transition, Susan has helped develop and directs a weekly support group for women in her community who have babies under one year of age.

Susan's interest in helping others establish healthy life patterns extends beyond her nursing career. For 15 years she worked as a personal trainer, managing individualized exercise, dietary, and fitness programs for children, adolescents, and adults. Her commitment to teaching others the value of establishing and maintaining healthy patterns for life continues and overflows to her husband Mark and their two sons Mitchel and Jared.

Susan is a strong believer that positive eating and exercise patterns improve health, self-esteem, and energy levels, as well as reduce illness, disease, and weight problems. To create healthy patterns, parents need to acquire basic knowledge on nutrition and activity through simple and realistic instruction that can be applied to everyday life—hence the purpose of this book.

Acknowledgments

Thank you to the following people for their valued input and critique of this book prior to publication. Their comments and suggestions have served to support the importance of helping our children establish and enjoy healthy patterns for life.

Thomas Wilson, M.D., Pediatrician and Father

Jacque Park-Byrkit, M.S., R.D., Dietician and Mother

Douglas Hancock, Health Educator and Personal Trainer

Kristen Johnk, Preschool Teacher and Mother

Barb Parkes, Home Health Nurse and Mother

And thank you to Mark Garson, (my husband, father of our two boys, and professionally a Medical Technologist) for his contributions toward seeing this book through from concept to publication.

Introduction

The increasing occurrence of weight problems, sedentary lifestyles, and poor health plagues families everywhere. With a little perseverance, maintaining healthy weight, feeling good, being energetic, decreasing occurrence of disease, and living longer lives is something we can achieve.

Today, more than 60 percent of adults in the United States are considered overweight or obese. Chronic weight gain does not happen overnight—it occurs over a period of years, frequently beginning in early childhood. Years ago, it was the exception to see an obese child. This is no longer true—the number of overweight children is shocking. In the last couple of decades, the obesity rate for children ages 6 to 11 has nearly doubled, and the rate for adolescents has tripled.

The number of overweight individuals in this country has reached epidemic levels and related health problems have skyrocketed. Physicians are now routinely treating children for serious Type 2 diabetes and hypertension problems, rarely seen in children just a decade ago. Overweight children are more prone to psychological problems like low self-esteem and depression. And, there is no question about it, overweight children are most likely to become obese adults with an accompanying increase in the number of physical and mental issues that go along with the condition.

Many children eat poorly, but due to high metabolism, lack of calories consumed, or other factors they still maintain an acceptable body weight. These children are often considered lucky. It is true they avoid the mental anguish and physical struggle many overweight individuals encounter, but they are not free from harm.

All children, regardless of weight, who eat badly and do not exercise on a regular basis have increased chances of becoming overweight adults and encountering accompanying difficulties. We must remember, serious health issues can develop internally despite how we look externally. Negative lifestyle patterns that cause significant weight gain in some people and little to none in others have similar potential for creating life-threatening problems.

Establishing healthy eating and exercise patterns is important for everyone. This book teaches parents about basic nutrition, how to create active lifestyles, and how to reduce harmful and nonproductive behaviors. Whether children are heavy, average, or thin, establishing positive eating and exercise patterns will help them grow into active, confident, and healthy adults.

For the most part, parents choose whether they raise their children to be within healthy or unhealthy parameters. By setting appropriate eating and activity patterns for children, parents will be giving their children the gift of a healthier, happier life.

How to Use This Book

This book was created to help children develop healthy lifestyle patterns through proper diet and exercise. It applies the knowledge and wisdom I have acquired as a mother, pediatric nurse, and health and physical fitness advocate. To a certain degree, it is a collaborative effort with others in my professional work field (see preceding acknowledgments page) as I have sought confirmation from them on my theories and applications.

Pattern Setting for Childhood Health was purposefully designed for easy reading with a distinct absence of potentially confusing medical terminology. Recommended lifestyle patterns have been "child tested" by my own children and "field tested" by many of my patients and friends, all with positive results. Although positive patterns are not always easy or convenient to implement, the benefits are well worth the effort for parents interested in raising healthy and happy individuals.

As we all know, every child has unique characteristics and their own set of prevailing circumstances. What works for one child may not work the same for another. Recommendations, therefore, should be tailored to meet the needs of each individual child and family situation. Nothing is set in stone and as with other aspects of parenting, flexibility must be considered.

This book can be used as an "in-progress" working tool. While reading, parents may choose to highlight points or recommendations that can be initiated immediately. A list of such ideas can be made and posted in the kitchen or other common areas. The list can be referred to when grocery lists are made and while meals are being prepared. Once the list has been committed to memory and effective patterns have been established, it can be discarded. The book can then be reviewed for more recommendations to be initiated. The learning process is then repeated.

By making only several changes at a time, family members will not feel deprived or become overwhelmed. Over a period of time a feeling of satisfaction will be felt many times over, as more and more of these short-term goals are met.

Some parents may choose to only make a few minor changes in the diet and exercise patterns of their families. However, even then a few positive lifestyle changes are better than none at all.

Pattern Setting for Childhood Health will help parents learn how to choose healthy foods and activities for their children. Under no condition is it to be used in place of medical advice. Children must have check-ups at regular intervals as recommended by their physician.

Chapter 1

Habit Hazards

When children consume a healthy diet and maintain an active lifestyle, they usually receive a healthy body in return. The opposite also applies—when children consume unhealthy foods and lead a sedentary lifestyle, they receive an unhealthy body in return. Although the theory sounds simple, most parents will agree that it is not.

Lifestyle Choices

Unfortunately, many children do not consume proper nutrients and therefore do not supply their bodies with the components needed to be healthy and strong for life. It is like building a house with sugar cubes and icing. The house may stay intact and look beautiful for a period of time, but with daily stress and wear and tear it will begin falling apart until it completely crumbles. It makes much more sense to build a house out of quality materials so it will be stable, strong, and attractive for many decades.

Children with unhealthy diets will experience deterioration, as would a house built of sugar cubes. Sooner or later these children experience complications including:

- ♦ unstable energy levels
- ♦ weak bones and muscles
- ♦ slower healing of injuries
- ♦ slower recovery from illness
- ♦ inability to fight disease

These are just a few of many examples. The bottom line is, parents who want their children to live long and healthy lives need to supply them with quality nutrition.

Many medical conditions are directly related to diet. Some of them are very serious. Such conditions include:

- ♦ heart disease
- ♦ high blood pressure
- ♦ iron deficiency anemia
- ♦ intestinal problems
- ♦ weight problems
- ♦ tooth decay

The body depends on nutrition to survive. Without it, the body is compromised and may not function as well or last as long.

Diet affects how we look. Children who consume a healthy diet and exercise on a regular basis are more likely to have an increased amount of muscle and a decreased amount of body fat, which gives them attractive body tone. Children who consume an unhealthy diet and do not exercise are more likely to have excess body fat and much less muscle tone. These children may be thin or of average build, but appear untoned and out of shape. The reasons for leading a healthy lifestyle and avoiding unhealthy foods are endless.

Chubby Children

Many of today's children are already a part of the epidemic of overweight individuals sweeping the country. These unfortunate children are at increased risk of immediate health disorders including:

◆ kidney disease

◆ high blood pressure

◆ high cholesterol

◆ sleep apnea

◆ inflammation of the pancreas

◆ hip, knee, feet, and joint problems

The risk is not all physical. Overweight children may have fewer friends, have lower self-esteem, be more depressed, and take part in fewer extracurricular activities than thinner children.

Family history plays a role in creating overweight children. If parents are overweight, their children have a much greater chance of becoming overweight. Genetics is the part we cannot change at this point in time. Luckily, genetics is only a piece of the puzzle and not the sole determining factor that makes a person fat, thin, or fall somewhere between.

No matter what genetic code a person is born with, eating patterns greatly affect a person's weight. **Many people who are overweight have overweight children and it may have little to do with genetics. In many situations, parents are just passing their own bad eating habits on to their children.**

Lack of physical activity is the other major reason children become overweight. In the age of computers and television, many children get all the fun they think they need by just sitting in one spot. What they need are enforced time limitations on sedentary activities as well as teaching and reminding of all the fun games that can be played based on old-fashioned running and jumping.

Most people who have been overweight will agree body fat is very difficult to lose and keep off. It is easier and healthier not to put it on in the first place. **Children need to be taught prevention so they will not have to struggle with weight problems later in life.**

Children who have already become overweight need intervention now. The older children get, the more difficult negative patterns are to change. Also, as time passes, overweight children become more and more overweight. Once overweight children become obese adolescents or adults, much harm has already taken place.

Unnecessarily Obese

Obesity is defined as an abnormal amount of fat on the body that meets or exceeds 20 to 30 percent over an average weight for age, sex, and height. The number of obese children is increasing significantly. Obesity is not discriminatory—it affects most ethnic groups, and people of every socioeconomic status.

Childhood obesity is a multi-system disease with potentially devastating consequences, many of which warrant special medical attention. Systems most greatly affected are:

- cardiovascular
- endocrine
- musculoskeletal
- neurological
- psychosocial
- pulmonary
- renal

By the time obese children are in their teens, many have the beginnings of heart disease, diabetes, or both. **Obese children are at much greater risk of premature illness and death than thinner children.**

Treatment for obesity is difficult, slow, and often not successful at all. **Prevention is the answer.** This ultimately requires family involvement, taking in fewer calories, and leading an active lifestyle.

Unhealthy eating and activity patterns negatively affect individuals of all ages and in all weight categories. Without supplying the body with proper building blocks, it is less able to function efficiently and a wide variety of problems can occur.

Chapter 2

Starting from Scratch

During the first few years of children's lives, parents are in complete control of all food and drink consumed. This formative time is the perfect opportunity to feed children a large variety of healthy foods. There are two important reasons why parents should take full advantage of this time. First, children deserve nothing less than good nutrition. Second, the eating habits parents help develop lay down the groundwork for the rest of their children's lives. Establishing healthy eating patterns is one of the best things parents can ever do for their children.

Preference Development

Babies are born with definite taste preferences. These preferences are for foods that are sweet, salty, and contain fat. Unfortunately, these tastes exclude those needed to enjoy many healthy foods. **Healthy taste preferences must be developed over time.** To acquire a taste for healthy food, children must be frequently exposed to the flavors of such foods.

Children under three years old eat what they are fed, so it is easy to keep them on an optimal diet. **If they frequently eat healthy foods, that is what they become accustomed to, like, and expect.** Also, children who infrequently eat unhealthy foods usually do not develop constant cravings for them. On the other hand, children who excessively eat junk food such as processed foods, fast foods, sweets, and packaged snacks are more likely to expect and crave such foods. That is when it becomes a struggle to get children to eat healthy foods. It is very beneficial to start children on nutritious foods early in life and continue the pattern for years to come.

Solid Introductions

Development of eating patterns, in regard to table foods, may be started as early as four months of age. At this point, table food is mainly given for variety and to begin the process of teaching children how to eat solid foods.

Children one year old and younger cannot eat enough solid food to maintain normal growth and development—they should remain on breast milk or formula to obtain full nutritional requirements. Since breast milk and formula offer the best overall nutrition, other fluids should not be used to replace them. Parents are advised to check with their child's physician prior to starting children on solid foods of any kind.

A rule to remember is that parents decide on the foods served and children decide how much to eat. From the day children are born, their bodies tell them when they are hungry and when they are not. In the beginning, children use this biological mechanism as their intake guide. This mechanism is ideal and parents should not attempt to alter it. Children should be allowed to stop eating when they show signs they are no longer hungry. It is unfortunate many people have learned to ignore this natural mechanism and therefore overeat. Listening to one's own body should be encouraged.

Children should not be forced to eat things they do not like. Doing this makes mealtime stressful and children less willing to try new foods. Instead, parents can continue offering refused or untouched foods on different days until their children learn to like them.

Parents should encourage children to taste new or previously disliked foods. A taste usually means a swallow, but even when food is spit out it is briefly tasted, which is one step toward developing that particular food preference. Like adults, there are some days when children do not want to eat certain foods and they need to develop tastes for others.

Over a period of time, a variety of foods should be introduced for meals and snacks. Children, as well as adults, enjoy eating different tastes, colors, and textures. Serving identical foods day by day should be avoided. When this happens, children are likely to get used to eating the same things and develop adversity to trying unfamiliar foods. Eating many different foods supplies the body with a wider variety of nutrients as well.

Parents should limit giving children sweet treats after meals. Parents love to give their children things that make them smile, but excessive sweets are something children get used to and learn to expect and crave. When this occurs, children realize treats come after meals and may start refusing to eat their meals and whine, fuss, and cry for dessert. This turns mealtime into a stressful power struggle between parents and children. When children become accustomed to sweets after meals, habits and cravings get established that may never go away. Parents who want to give their children special treats are better off treating them to activities they enjoy, like going for walks or reading books together.

Setting the Stage

When establishing eating patterns, it is most beneficial to involve the whole family. Anyone preparing food should be educated on which foods to purchase and serve, and how to prepare meals.

When possible, families should eat together. Family members have the first and most lasting influence on children. Children look at parents and older siblings to see how eating is supposed to be done.

Parents should display role-model behaviors children can learn from, and parents should not forget that what is eaten and not eaten will get noticed. Family meals should take place in a positive atmosphere. It does not always work out, but parents should attempt to make mealtime a calm, unhurried, and enjoyable experience. Reminding children to eat is fine, but parents need to try to avoid stressful lectures about eating. Mealtimes should be happy times with family—this helps to create a positive disposition in all family members, and children develop better eating habits.

Parents should resist the temptation to lecture or scold about eating. Prompting is fine, but it must be in a positive manner. Children should be praised for things like trying different foods, using good manners, and making adequate food choices. It is not a good idea to praise children for things like cleaning their plate, eating all of their food, or eating a lot. This makes children think the goal is to eat amounts that make parents happy and they may ignore that their body feels as if it has had enough food.

Most adults have a weakness for certain foods. Usually they are sweet, high-fat, or salty treats that should not be eaten on a regular basis. When parents want to indulge, they should do so when children are not present. **Parents should not let their junk food cravings become their children's junk food cravings.**

Appetites come and go during different stages of development. Sometimes children have drastic changes in eating patterns from day to day or month to month. This is normal as long as children gain weight and develop properly. Parents who feel their children are not eating normal amounts should consult their child's physician for advice.

Chapter 3

Pattern Setting, Plain and Simple

Negative patterns in children are usually set because parents do not know any differently, or because parents choose to take what appears to be the easiest and least stressful route. This is understandable during the periods of high stress and low energy that come with raising children. Unfortunately, negative patterns end up increasing stress in the long run, because unhealthy or annoying habits created may remain for a very long time.

Pattern setting happens whether parents realize it or not. Prior to allowing actions to become patterns, parents need to decide which patterns are mutually beneficial for each child and the family as a whole. **It is important that parents do not start anything they do not want continued, because patterns that become established may be harmful and very difficult to break.**

Productive Patterns

Pattern setting begins soon after birth as infants fall into patterns for everyday activities like sleeping and eating. It is advisable for parents to guide behaviors into desired directions to achieve certain outcomes. To do this successfully, parents need to agree on what will be achieved and decide which steps will be taken to reach such goals.

> **For example:** Babies can be taught to routinely go to bed and sleep without a bottle. To achieve this goal with the least difficulty, parents should avoid putting children in their cribs with a bottle. (If the pattern of sleeping with a bottle never begins, it does not become a habit that has to be broken.) Babies at least eight weeks old (younger babies usually fall asleep while being held and fed) should have on a clean, dry diaper and temperature-appropriate clothing. Parents can relax babies by sitting in a darkened room, singing lullabies, rocking, or quietly telling stories with their baby in their arms. If they are hungry, breast feeding or bottle feeding is advisable. When babies become very sleepy, but are not yet asleep, they should be placed in their cribs and left alone. Parents should frequently check on their babies. Those who cry can be gently touched for reassurance, but should not be picked up. After several nights of this, babies learn the pattern and go to sleep without a bottle.

This example teaches children that after all needs are met, the pattern is to become relaxed, go to bed, then fall asleep.

There are many benefits to establishing this pattern. When children wake up during the night, they can get themselves back to sleep without the help of a parent or bottle. This saves children, parents, and other family members from unnecessary heartache, frustration, and lost sleep. It also teaches children exactly what the crib is to be used for—sleep. Pattern setting takes some extra work in the beginning stages, but once patterns are established, the work is over and everyone benefits.

Nonproductive Patterns

Some parents choose not to consciously guide behaviors into certain directions, and they let children fall into their own patterns.

> **For example:** Parents may decide to put their babies to bed with a bottle and let them drink to relax themselves. This seems like the easy way out, and at first it really can be. It frees parents up to do other things while their children drink from their bottles and fall asleep. This becomes a problem when children associate having a bottle with going to sleep and have difficulty going to sleep without one. When this occurs, children either cry until they get a bottle or cry themselves to sleep.

Putting babies to bed with a bottle sets patterns that make them feel they need a bottle in order to relax and go to sleep. This also applies when they wake up during the night—they frequently cry each time they awaken because they do not know how to calm themselves and go back to sleep on their own. This disrupts the process of developing good sleep patterns. Another problem with developing this pattern is that children who sleep with bottles in their mouths are prone to cavities in newly erupting teeth.

Parental Payoff

Patterns are an important part of childhood development. They teach children they can count on things repeatedly occurring in similar ways. Through this process, children grow to realize certain individuals can be trusted to fulfill their needs. Children who have positive daily patterns often feel more confident, calm, and secure about their surroundings.

Chapter 4

Patterns for Safety

Child safety should be a top priority for every parent. Offering age-appropriate foods, preventing unsafe mealtime activities, and introducing new foods slowly and cautiously are all necessary to keep children out of dietary danger.

Dangerous Delectables

Children of all ages are at risk for choking. Prior to starting young children on table foods, parents need to have a clear understanding of what is safe for them to eat and what is not. Parents must completely avoid giving young children food they could choke on including:

- ♦ hot dogs
- ♦ fruit with pits
- ♦ grapes
- ♦ whole beans
- ♦ hard candies
- ♦ jellybeans
- ♦ chewing gum
- ♦ nuts and seeds
- ♦ popcorn
- ♦ marshmallows

Small round foods like these are very dangerous because they fit perfectly into the airway and can cause an occlusion. Food must always be cut up into small, irregular-shaped, bite-sized pieces.

Big globs of peanut butter must not be given to young children either—peanut butter can obstruct a child's airway. Parents can check with their child's physician at each visit to obtain current lists of recommended, age-appropriate foods to try and hazardous foods to avoid.

Mealtime Monitoring

Choking risk applies not only to what children eat, but also where they eat. All children should be seated while eating and younger children need to be closely observed at all times. Children should not be allowed to walk, run, jump, lie down, or play while eating. Excessive activity and laughter with food in the mouth can cause choking. Setting a pattern that children always eat at the dinner table is helpful. It is safer and keeps the messes in one spot.

Allergy Awareness

Any food can cause an allergic response. Reactions are most likely to occur within 24 hours of eating a new food. It is advisable to introduce new foods to children one at a time and wait a day or two before introducing another. Then if a reaction occurs, parents have a good chance of determining which new food may have caused the reaction.

Certain foods have a much higher risk of causing reactions than other foods do. Such foods should not be introduced to very young children. Examples of these foods are eggs, which should not be introduced prior to one year of age, and peanut butter, which should not be introduced prior to two years of age.

Food allergies can be inherited and children with other allergic conditions are more prone to them. Until parents are sure their children are not prone to allergies, they should be extra careful to introduce new foods very slowly. If parents see anything unusual in a child's appearance or behavior, the child's physician or 911 should be called immediately.

Chapter 5

Simply Colorful

Children as well as adults should eat a wide variety of foods each day. Sounds simple, right? Well, actually, most people struggle with this concept and have many questions. How much variety is recommended? Which foods are best? How much of each food should be eaten?

Few parents have a degree in nutrition, nor are they able to take time out of their busy schedules to study up on the topic. Luckily this is not necessary—my philosophy is to make it simple.

When planning daily meals and snacks, each different food should be a different color. The more colors consumed throughout the day the better—that's it. A wide variety of color offers the widest variety of nutrients. Here are some fruits and vegetables that can add color to any plate:

Blue, Purple, and Black

blueberries, cherries, purple grapes, plums, purple cabbage, black beans, blackberries, raisins

Green

peas, spinach, broccoli, zucchini, avocado, green bell peppers, asparagus, romaine lettuce, honeydew melon, kiwi fruit, artichokes, brussel sprouts, green apples, green pears, green beans, green cabbage, cucumbers, celery

Orange

apricots, nectarines, peaches, carrots, sweet potatoes, yams, pumpkin, mango, cantaloupe, oranges, papaya, tangerines

Red or Pink

tomatoes, strawberries, raspberries, watermelon, guava, pink grapefruit, cherries, blood oranges, cranberries, rhubarb, radishes, red apples, beets, red onion, red bell peppers, pomegranates

Yellow

yellow bell peppers, squash, bananas, pineapple, yellow pears, corn, yellow apples, grapefruit

White and Brown

potatoes, white peaches, cauliflower, jicama, parsnips, turnips, onions, dates, figs, mushrooms, ginger root, brown pears

Nutritional needs vary from person to person depending on age, sex, stage of life, and activity level. Eating a variety of healthy food increases the chance of obtaining adequate nutrients.

Chapter 6

Basics Made Simple

Most people have seen a diagram of the Food Pyramid. It is an excellent teaching tool for health class, but few adults can correctly recall the suggested intake percentages for each food group. Even if we all remembered, would we take the time to figure out the daily intake amounts every day for each member of the family? Many families are short on time and long on stress, therefore, we can simplify.

All parents need to do to guarantee their families receive a well-rounded nutrition balance is to learn the following food types, keep a mental note of how much each should be consumed each day, and apply the knowledge to everyday life.

Most

Fruits, Vegetables, Whole grains

Moderate

(Protein)
Milk products, Legumes, Fish, Poultry, Soy, Lean meat, Eggs

Few

Fats, Sugars

These amounts can vary from meal to meal as long as by the end of each day, family members have consumed many different fruits, vegetables, and whole grains; a moderate amount of protein; and only a small amount of fat and sugar.

Parents can use this simple tool to help decide food amounts when preparing and serving family meals and snacks. Planning meals will become easier, and parents no longer have to wonder if they are serving their families appropriate amounts of each food group.

Chapter 7

Wonderful Water

The human body is 50 to 75 percent water, with children's bodies containing the higher percentages. Water affects every organ in the body and plays a significant role in life and maintaining good health. Water facilitates many vital body functions such as:

- allowing blood to flow, carrying nutrients to and from cells throughout the body
- transporting waste out of the body through urine, feces, perspiration, and respiration
- cooling the body
- helping the brain do its job more efficiently
- lubricating joints and muscles
- softening skin
- preventing constipation

Early Introductions

Breast-fed babies get all the water they need through breast milk, so they do not need to consume water until they are weaned from breast feeding. Formula-fed babies may or may not get enough water from formula. They may need small amounts of water each day to maintain proper hydration.

Excess water should not be given to babies who are underweight or who have difficulty maintaining weight because it may fill them up and replace needed calories. In these cases, a physician's guidance is necessary.

Frequent water consumption is a great pattern to begin during early childhood. Prior to a child's first birthday, parents should introduce water. Some young children will immediately like it, while others will not. Either way, parents should continue offering water daily. If it is continually being refused, parents can try offering it when children are most thirsty. If water is the only option, most children will drink it. Some children may be more inclined to drink water if they have a special cup or bottle that is colorful and fun to drink out of. The trick is to never fill the special cup or bottle with anything other than water.

Planned Preferences

Parents may choose to establish certain patterns around when water is served and when other drinks are allowed.

> **For example:** Parents may choose to always serve water with lunch and dinner. Other parents may choose to serve other healthy beverages with meals, but allow only water at other times during the day. Whatever pattern parents create will become the accepted routine.

If parents consistently offer water every day, children will usually get used to it and may even grow to prefer it to other drinks. Children who drink water regularly will probably continue to drink it for the rest of their lives—whereas children who drink only sweet drinks will likely never develop a taste for water.

People who drink sugary drinks instead of water consume a lot of sugar and many extra calories. This alone can lead to significant weight gain. Water is the best drink for the body—it contains no sugar, artificial sweeteners, fat, or calories. Children who drink water have a definite health benefit over those who do not.

Handy Hydration

Drinking water is inexpensive, readily available, and convenient. It can be taken just about anywhere by placing it into a diaper bag or backpack. Unlike soda and juice, water can be taken into cars or public places without fears of messes or stains from spills that may occur. Also unlike other drinks, it does not go bad when unrefrigerated and is still palatable at room temperature. Keeping water handy while out of the house is a great way to avoid purchasing expensive sugary beverages and gets children used to the idea of drinking water to satisfy thirst.

Chapter 8

Breakfast First

Many families have more commitments than they have time. Because preparing and eating healthy breakfasts can be time-consuming, it is common for both adults and children to skip it completely or grab something on the run. **There are many areas in which families can compromise in order to save time, but breakfast should not be one of them.** A nutritious breakfast is essential for starting each day.

Some people like to eat as soon as they awaken, while others like to wait a couple of hours. Whatever the preference, eating breakfast should be made a priority. Parents can choose, or help children choose, foods that provide energy and good nutrition that can be eaten at a convenient time. Foods containing whole grains along with a little protein will keep energy levels up, brains working, and stomachs from rumbling for several hours. Breakfasts should be fairly low in fat and sugar. Seeing that children eat healthy breakfasts is an important part of parenting.

Productive Planning

Breakfast may sound completely impossible for families who rush around all morning and run out the door without a minute to spare. These families can work together to discover alternative plans.

> **For example:** One member of the family can get up 15 minutes earlier than the rest of the family—age-appropriate family members can take turns doing this. While other family members sleep, the early bird prepares a quick, nutritious breakfast for them. When everyone else gets up, breakfast is ready. Family members, other than the early bird, spend no time preparing or waiting for breakfast to be served—they just sit down and eat. If family members like to eat while commuting to their destination or eat later in the morning, breakfast can be prepared in the same fashion and packaged up to be taken along.
>
> For those family members who can not bear the thought of getting up any earlier than they have to, breakfast can be prepared the night before. It can be stored in the refrigerator overnight then heated in a microwave as needed.

Family members can brainstorm to come up with options that might work for their individual situations.

Outstanding Options

Following are a few suggestions for healthy breakfasts that are quick and easy—many of them can be prepared in advance and some can be eaten while on the run:

- egg-substitute vegetable omelet and whole-wheat toast (omelets can be made small and stuck between the toast for tasty sandwiches to go)
- low-fat cottage cheese topped with cut-up fresh fruit or unsweetened applesauce
- peanut butter sandwich on whole-wheat bread and a piece of fresh fruit
- low-fat and low-sugar trail mix made at home with a mixture of several dry cereals, raisins and other dried fruit, nuts and seeds, or whatever else taste buds desire (for those who are age-appropriate)
- bran or whole-wheat muffin (low-fat and low-sugar) and a banana
- whole-wheat bagel with low-fat cream cheese and tomato
- whole-wheat French toast or waffle topped with fresh fruit and served with scrambled egg substitute
- oatmeal topped with dried or fresh fruit and skim milk
- low-fat, low-sugar cereal topped with fruit (add low-fat milk or yogurt)

Just Junk

Food manufacturers are well aware of the desire for foods that are quick and convenient. There are literally hundreds of products on the market that fit this description and many of them are eaten for breakfast. Unfortunately, most of these foods are low on nutrients, full of fat and sugar, and are definitely not advisable for breakfast. Below are some examples of frequently eaten foods that are not healthy meal alternatives:

- doughnuts
- toaster pastries
- sugary cereals
- anything fried
- white flour pancakes or waffles
- sweet, white flour muffins
- fast food breakfasts

Treats are fine but they should be limited to a little each day, and breakfast is not the time for such treats. Overnight, our bodies go many hours without food. In the morning we are depleted of energy and must refuel. People who skip breakfast or replenish with junk food are doing their bodies a great disservice.

People who eliminate breakfast altogether in order to reduce calories usually end up getting overdepleted and eating more calories over the course of the day than they otherwise would. It takes effort and commitment to serve family members nutritious breakfasts, but in a short time eating a variety of healthy foods will be a beneficial part of the daily routine the whole family can enjoy.

Chapter 9

Vibrant Vegetables

Vegetables help nourish the body so it is healthy, strong, and functions properly. Vegetables generally are high in vitamins, minerals, and antioxidants. These nutrients help create and maintain healthy skin, glands, eye function, and a strong immune system. They help the body fight various illnesses and can even help fight cancer and other diseases.

Vegetables contain folic acid, which is essential for normally functioning cells and blood. Vegetables also contain fiber that helps digestion. People who eat adequate amounts of fiber are less likely to have serious bowel problems or heart disease, or to become obese. It is important we provide vegetables for our children to keep them as healthy as they can be.

Reaching Recommended Requirements

It is recommended that children have two or three servings of vegetables each day. Unfortunately, many people, young and old, do not consume daily requirements. Some people do not eat them at all. Frequently, parents who do not like vegetables will not serve many of them to their children. Because these children do not eat adequate amounts of vegetables, or see their role models eating them, they usually never become fond of them either. This is terrible. **If children do not learn to eat vegetables early in life, they may never really develop a taste for them and may choose not to eat them later in life.** There are so many different kinds of vegetables—parents should be able to find at least a few different "tastes" family members can enjoy.

Ideally, parents start children on vegetables during the baby-food stage, then move into softly steamed vegetables that are smashed up and spoon fed. If children eat them when they first begin on solids, they are less likely to develop a negative attitude toward them. Since children learn by watching what parents do, parents should set good examples and eat a wide variety of vegetables too.

When preparing vegetables for young children, parents must make sure all hard vegetables are cooked to be very soft, and cut up into small pieces. Small round vegetables, like peas and beans, can be inhaled or cause choking, so they should be smashed or not served to young children.

Veggie Variety

Vegetables are an excellent way to add color and nutrition to any plate of food. Unfortunately, many parents tend to repeatedly buy and prepare the same two or three types. This gets monotonous for everyone in the family, so the vegetables may not be eaten. The trick is to buy a wide variety of them. Parents then can serve the same ones less frequently. This way everyone gets more variety and nutrients in their diet and families do not get bored with repetition.

A nice way to discover new vegetables is to walk through the grocery store's produce, frozen food, and canned food sections and take an inventory of what is available. Consider all vegetables, even those never tried or previously disliked. Chances are, plenty of vegetables will be found that family members will enjoy and benefit from.

Food processing sometimes changes the nutrients of food. Fresh and frozen vegetables undergo little or no processing, so they usually contain the most vitamins and minerals. They also have little or no added salt. Generous portions of fresh and thawed frozen vegetables can be added to any meal or enjoyed alone as nutritional snacks throughout the day.

Canned vegetables have to be processed for preservation. During processing, salt is added. Fortunately, much of the salt is actually in the canning fluid that can simply be discarded. To further reduce salt intake, vegetables can be rinsed in water prior to eating. Canned vegetables can be very convenient since they can sit on shelves for months, and are quick and easy to prepare. It is advisable to buy fresh, frozen, and canned vegetables so there is always a variety to choose from.

Salad Savvy

Raw vegetables are often most nutritious. Some adults eat salads frequently, but do not feed them to their children. Salads are not just an adult food. Children of all ages can enjoy salads when they are made from combinations of age-appropriate vegetables. Young children can be introduced to salads as finger food. Vegetable choices for them might include:

- ◆ diced tomatoes
- ◆ sliced olives
- ◆ pre-cooked broccoli, cauliflower, and carrots
- ◆ canned green beans
- ◆ canned beets
- ◆ baby corn

Young children love colors and textures, and instinct tells them to discover objects by putting them in their mouths. This is what makes it so easy to get them to eat vegetables at this stage.

Older children who have a full set of teeth can be served raw vegetables including:

◆ broccoli	◆ sliced bell peppers
◆ cucumbers	◆ zucchini
◆ cauliflower	◆ celery
◆ baby carrots	◆ jicama

Raw vegetables are great for lunch, dinner, or snacks. They are perfect for hungry, fussy children who have a difficult time waiting for meals to be prepared. Serving vegetables before meals helps children get their daily requirements, and are not usually heavy enough to spoil children's appetites. When mealtime rolls around, parents can relax, knowing that some vegetables have already been eaten—of course, they can always have more with the meal!

Preparation Possibilities

Steaming is one of the healthiest ways vegetables can be prepared. Some people prefer steamed vegetables to raw because they are easier to eat and digest. Another benefit is they can be prepared quickly and easily on the stove or in the microwave.

Many people choose to boil their vegetables, but this is not the ideal way to cook them. Some of the vitamins and minerals are lost into the water and discarded when boiled vegetables are drained. Overcooking often occurs when vegetables are boiled—this causes even more nutrients to be lost.

Children like finger foods of all types, especially when dipped in sauces. Serving vegetables with dip is fine on occasion, but they should be served plain as well. When served raw, children will learn to like the flavor of vegetables instead of unhealthy sauces, dips, or dressings. When children refuse to eat vegetables or simply do not eat enough of them, parents can be creative.

Raw vegetables can be chopped or grated and added to sandwiches or foods like potato salad and pasta salad. Cooked vegetables can be topped with spaghetti sauce or sprinkled with a little cheese. They can also be added to many main dishes like macaroni and cheese, spaghetti, soups, and stews. Extra tomato-based sauce and vegetables can be added to pizza. Parents can evaluate favorite family recipes, and one or two vegetables can probably be added to each dish without anyone disapproving.

Chapter 10

Fantastic Fruit

Fruits are similar to vegetables in that they provide many essential vitamins and minerals that keep us healthy and help our bodies fight and prevent illness and disease. Fruit is also one of the best sources of vitamin C, which is necessary for good health. Fruit is a healthy and convenient food most children naturally like and gladly eat.

Variables for Variety

Children should eat two or three servings of fruit a day. Because most children like fruit and frequently eat it when it is offered, daily requirements are usually met without difficulty. Unfortunately, less-healthy versions of fruit are often served to children, so many of them consume excess sugar and additives. It is essential that parents not only serve the recommended amount of fruit to their children, but that they also make proper fruit choices.

Fruits come in many different colors, textures, shapes, and sizes. Fresh or unsweetened frozen fruits are generally the healthiest choices. Canned fruit in natural juices is acceptable, but parents should try to avoid serving canned fruit in heavy or light syrup—these contain a lot of sugar and have substantially more calories.

Dried fruit is usually a very nutritious alternative to whole fruit; however, labels should be read because some dried fruits contain added sweeteners. Dried fruits are high in calories so children who are overweight should be limited to a couple of pieces of whole, dried fruit per day. Because the body receives the most nutrients when a variety of fruits are consumed, it is advisable that parents keep fresh, canned, and dried fruit on hand.

Whole fruit is much better for the body than fruit juice is. Whole fruit is more filling, contains much less sugar, and provides fiber. Whether fruit juice beverages contain 5% real juice or 100% real juice, they contain a lot of sugar and calories. Offering juice to fulfill daily requirements of fruit is not recommended.

Produce Pesticides

Fruits and vegetables purchased at grocery stores are very likely to contain pesticides, so all fresh produce that is not home-grown should be washed or peeled. Even produce labeled "pesticide-free" may contain chemicals.

Some chemicals are oil-based and do not rinse off completely with just water. When possible, a very small amount of dish soap can be used to further remove pesticide residue. Since chemicals may be harmful, it is best to be cautious and eliminate unnecessary consumption.

Chapter 11

Great Grains

Grains are carbohydrates. Carbohydrates are broken down into sugar, which is a major source of energy for the body. Some types of carbohydrates are very nutritious while others are not. Unfortunately, many children eat an excess of unhealthy carbohydrates and not enough of the healthy ones. A simple explanation and comparison of different products may make it easier for families to make healthier choices.

Completely Complex

Complex carbohydrates are great for the body and should supply more than half of the total calories consumed each day. Examples of complex carbohydrates include whole-grain breads, brown rice, whole-grain pasta, and whole-grain cereals.

Complex carbohydrates are slowly broken down into sugar and slowly released into the bloodstream. This provides a constant supply of energy for several hours. Because fiber in complex carbohydrates slows absorption, the stomach feels full longer. Whole grains have more flavor than processed grains and are naturally low in fat.

Simply Sugar

The other type of carbohydrates are called simple carbohydrates. These foods supply a large amount of sugar and sometimes a lot of fat. Examples of these foods include white bread, white rice, and sweets like cookies and pastries. Simple carbohydrates contain little or no nutritional value. Some people eat simple carbohydrates in place of foods high in vitamins and minerals. This provides calories without providing adequate nutrients.

Unlike complex carbohydrates, simple carbohydrates—when eaten alone—are broken down into sugar that is released into the bloodstream very quickly. This release triggers a very rapid elevation in blood sugar. The body receives a jolt of quick energy, then blood sugar drops and the body experiences low energy and often excessive hunger. At this point individuals are likely to seek out more food, and more food means even more calories.

Consuming large amounts of simple carbohydrates should be avoided, but a moderate amount is acceptable. When carbohydrates of any kind are eaten, it is better to include them with a mixed meal. Protein and dietary fat slow breakdown and absorption, which minimizes blood-sugar fluctuations and rebound hunger.

Better Breads

There are many bread types to choose from but none are as nutritious as 100% whole-wheat and 100% whole-grain varieties. The reason for this has to do with flour processing.

Wheat and grain are ground to make whole-wheat and whole-grain flour. This flour is a complex carbohydrate and is the most healthy and natural state of flour. This flour is used to bake whole-wheat and whole-grain breads.

Many people like white bread, so white flour is created. In order to do this, healthy whole-wheat and whole-grain flour is bleached and processed. This removes nutrients from the grain and changes it into a simple carbohydrate. Manufacturers often add synthetic vitamins to white flour, which is otherwise nutrient-poor. The product is then called *enriched flour*. To state it simply, **100% whole-wheat and 100% whole-grain breads are naturally very nutritious, whereas white breads are not.**

Labels on breads can be deceiving. Many people think they are making adequate choices, when they really are not. There are so many different bread types on the market it becomes difficult to determine what is what.

The easiest way to make healthy bread choices is by reading the front of the packaging. Such labeling should always read "100% whole-wheat" or "100% whole-grain." When those exact words are not printed, bread will usually contain primarily white flour. When in doubt, the ingredient list can simply be read.

The first ingredient of the healthiest breads will always be whole-wheat or whole-grain flour. Ingredient labels that begin with the terms *flour*, *enriched flour*, or *wheat flour* tell the consumer the bread is made primarily with white flour.

Bread manufacturers make white bread with a small amount of whole-wheat flour added and fool consumers by calling it wheat bread. Some companies even add caramel coloring to make wheat bread look darker so people think it is healthier. **Wheat bread is not whole-wheat bread.**

Changing bread is one of the easiest transitions that can be made toward healthier eating. **The key to remember is the front of the packaging should always say "100% whole-wheat" or "100% whole-grain," and the first ingredient listed should include the words *whole-wheat* or *whole-grain*.**

Rice Recommendations

Brown rice contains many more vitamins and minerals than other types of rice do. It is also full of fiber so it keeps the stomach full for hours and aids in digestion. As with flour, rice can be processed and bleached—the end product is nutrient-poor white rice. This process also changes the complex carbohydrate (brown rice) into a simple carbohydrate (white rice).

There are many types of rice on the market and most are just variations of white rice. Brown rice comes in long and short grain. Whatever the preference, **packaging must read "brown rice."** It is just that simple.

Some people mistake fried rice (served in restaurants) for brown rice. Indeed it is brown, but only from adding brown soy sauce to white rice during the frying process. Few restaurants serve brown rice, because it cannot be made in just a few minutes like white rice can. Also, many people are content eating the less healthy variety, so few request brown rice. Some restaurants precook brown rice and heat it up for those who request it.

Making the switch to brown rice is another simple change parents can make that will do their families a world of good.

Preferably Pasta

Pasta is one of the most frequently prepared family foods. It is quick and children love it. Pasta can be purchased that is made with either white or 100% whole-grain flour. Just like with bread, **pasta made from 100% whole-grain is a complex carbohydrate and is very healthy, while pasta made from white flour is a simple carbohydrate and provides few nutrients.**

White pasta is inexpensive and stocked in mass quantities on grocer's shelves. This makes it very easy for parents to stock the family pantry and serve it frequently. White pasta comes in a large variety of shapes and sizes. It is also used in boxed macaroni and pasta dishes, as well as in frozen dinners. These meal choices are quick and easy to prepare but low on nutrition. Meals prepared with white pasta can be served now and then, but it is not advisable to serve them frequently.

For healthy alternatives to boxed white pasta meals, parents can purchase whole-wheat versions of boxed macaroni and cheese from health-food stores. These provide more nutrients, taste great, and are quick to prepare. Whole-grain pastas topped with various low-fat sauces are also healthy options.

Restaurants usually serve white pasta because it is more convenient and most people do not request otherwise. Families who eat out infrequently may choose to splurge and have white pasta during these times. A positive step toward serving more nutritious meals is to change from white to whole-wheat pasta at least half the time.

Smart Cereal Selections

Cereal is something children usually love. It is a very nutritious meal or snack when the right types are chosen. **Parents need to look for cereals that contain high-fiber grains—like whole wheat, whole bran, and oats—with only small amounts of added sugar and other sweeteners.** Nutritious choices will usually be dark brown and some will have visible nuts and grains. These cereals are packed with vitamins, minerals, and fiber and are low in sugar and salt. Other than granola that has oil added to it, they are usually low in fat. Parents should read labels and decide which cereals they want their family members to eat.

The majority of cereals on grocery store shelves are marketed toward children through fancy commercials and colorful boxes with prizes inside. These cereals are usually simple carbohydrates with excessive amounts of sugar. In other words, they are junk food.

Synthetic vitamins are added to junk food cereals, which makes the nutritional facts listed on boxes look impressive at a glance, but parents should not be fooled.

Young children should be started off on healthy cereals and not introduced to the sugary variety at all. When children become older and learn of sugary cereals from other sources, parents can explain that sugary cereals are not good for them. Children who want to try other cereals can help parents decide on healthy alternatives.

Children who are already used to sugary cereals may be difficult to persuade. In those situations, when sugary cereals run out they should be replaced with healthy cereal. Children can go to the grocery store and help parents choose which cereals to try. If children play a part in the decision-making process, they may be more eager to try something new. Dried or fresh fruit may be added when children desire sweeter-tasting cereals, but sugary cereals themselves should remain on grocer's shelves.

Maintaining Moderation

Many foods like cookies, cake, doughnuts, muffins, pastries, white pizza crust, and most desserts fall into the simple carbohydrate category. Most of these products are made with white flour, white sugar, and shortening; therefore, they have little nutritional value and are very high in sugar and fat. They should be consumed only very infrequently.

People who choose not to give up favorite snack foods can shop for healthier varieties at health-food shops, bakeries, and specialty shops. Such treats can also be made by scratch using whole-wheat flour and minimal amounts of oil, butter, shortening, and sugar. Avoiding simple-carbohydrate snack foods completely may not be realistic, but keeping consumption to a minimum is an obtainable goal.

Chapter 12

Fabulous Fiber

Fiber is the indigestible part of plant foods. It is a complex carbohydrate that is often referred to as roughage. Fiber is the part of fruits and vegetables that is not digested or absorbed. Even though it does not provide vitamins, minerals, or calories, it is an important part of a healthy diet.

The benefits of fiber include:

♦ regulating blood sugar and cholesterol levels

♦ aiding digestion

♦ promoting normal bowel movements

♦ helping to prevent many diseases

Through some of these processes, fiber can reduce the risk of some cancers. Fiber is obviously an important part of any healthy eating regimen.

Smooth Passage

The two types of fiber are called soluble and insoluble. Soluble fiber absorbs and holds fluid and performs the following functions:

♦ slows digestion and the rate of nutrient absorption from the stomach and intestines

♦ controls blood-sugar levels so they remain steady

♦ absorbs a portion of consumed fat and passes it as waste instead of allowing it to be absorbed into the bloodstream

Soluble fiber is naturally low in saturated fat. It contains no cholesterol and may even help cholesterol levels from becoming high, which protects against cardiovascular disease. It is also helpful in preventing weight gain.

Foods that contain soluble fiber include:

♦ vegetables

♦ fruits

♦ dried beans and peas

♦ oats, rice, bran, barley, and grains

Clean Sweep

Insoluble fiber absorbs fluid in the colon and adds bulk and softness to stools. This keeps stools moving and intestines cleaned out, which helps protect the body from colon cancer. Insoluble fiber also may help prevent constipation, diverticulosis, and hemorrhoids.

Foods that contain insoluble fiber include:

♦ plant leaves

♦ fruit

♦ vegetable skins and peels

Where there is fiber, there usually will be vitamins and minerals. Plant foods and whole-grain products that are high in fiber contain many nutrients. Ways to increase fiber intake include:

♦ eating vegetables and fruits with the skins on

♦ eating fresh and dried fruit

♦ eating a variety of beans

♦ eating dark green lettuce or spinach

Fiber is great for the body as long as intake is not in excess. Consumption should be spread out during the course of the day, and fiber supplementation should not be done unless ordered by a physician. If large amounts of fiber are consumed at one time, gas with stomach bloating and constipation, or diarrhea may occur.

Fluid consumption is important with fiber consumption because fluid helps fiber do its job. Fiber without adequate fluid can cause constipation and discomfort. A healthy diet including adequate amounts of fluid and fiber helps build and maintain healthy bodies.

Chapter 13

Magnificent Milk Products

Milk products are excellent sources of calcium, which is needed for bone growth and repair. They are also great sources of protein, which helps the body build, repair, and maintain tissues. Calcium and protein needs differ during one's life span. The need is highest during stages of rapid growth, which is why children of all ages benefit from milk products.

It is recommended children consume at least two or three servings of milk products each day. Milk products include milk, yogurt, cheese, cottage cheese, and ice cream. It is wise to offer a variety of these products throughout the day.

Age-Appropriate Provisions

Children may have milk products when they begin eating table foods, with the exception of cow's milk. Milk should not be given to children until they become one year old. Although breast milk, formula, and cow's milk contain similar amounts of fat and calories, cow's milk contains three times the amount of protein that breast milk and formula do. This quantity of protein is too high for children under one year. Diluting cow's milk is not an option, because it would not contain enough fat and calories for proper nutrition.

Another problem with feeding cow's milk to children under the age of one is that it does not contain enough iron to meet nutritional requirements. Children who are switched to milk too soon can become anemic. Young children are also more prone to allergies than older children, and cow's milk may cause a reaction. Therefore, the best fluids for children under one year of age are breast milk and formula.

When the time comes to introduce cow's milk to children, it is advisable to stick with plain white milk. Adding flavors to milk increases sugar intake and conditions desire for sweeter foods. Most people find milk has a wonderful taste and does not need added flavors to make it enjoyable.

Children frequently like yogurt because it is creamy and sweet. Parents like serving it because it is nutritious. In addition to calcium and protein, yogurt contains beneficial active cultures. These active cultures may cause a temporary upset in the gastrointestinal tract of young children. As with any new food, children should be started with modest amounts to make sure it is well tolerated.

Older children can enjoy yogurt as desired with meals or snacks. Children who tend to overindulge in foods should be limited on flavored yogurt consumption because it contains moderate amounts of sweetener. As with many foods, a serving or two is beneficial but consuming large amounts should be avoided.

Milk products can be purchased in many different fat and calorie contents. Children between the ages of one and two should be fed whole milk and full-fat milk products. Fat consumption is important during infancy and early childhood, because it helps the brain develop properly. Obtaining fats from healthy sources that add more nutrients is preferable to those from unhealthy sources with little or no nutritional value.

Young children who are overweight may be put on reduced-fat dairy products with their physician's approval. Because low-fat and high-fat dairy varieties contain similar nutrients, few children over the age of two need to consume products with higher fat.

Transition Time

Some milk products can be purchased in lower-fat varieties without children noticing any change. This may or may not be the case with milk. Children who have become accustomed to drinking whole milk may resist drastic changes such as suddenly changing to skim milk. For these children, changing from whole milk to 2% milk is a step in the right direction. Over time, parents can purchase milk with less and less fat until skim or 1% milk is palatable.

Once family members are used to low-fat versions of dairy products, a healthy pattern is set. Consuming low-fat dairy products instead of higher-fat varieties can save thousands of fat grams and extra calories over a period of time. **Changing to low-fat dairy products is highly recommended when extra fat and calories are no longer needed.**

Pure Pastures

Many commercial cows are currently given genetically engineered growth hormone. The injections are said to carry many benefits, the main one being that it helps farmers produce more milk and remain profitable. The use and safety of these substances is very controversial.

The use of synthetic hormones in commercial cows has been widely tested over the last couple of decades, and milk produced under such conditions has been proven safe for human consumption. Due to these facts, hormone use in cows has FDA (Food and Drug Administration) approval, and at this time no special labeling is required.

Many individuals are not convinced these so-called agricultural advances are safe. They question unknown long-term effects on humans as well as cancer-causing possibilities of consumed synthetic substances. Increased infection rates and suppressed immune systems in these cows are also points of concern, since antibiotics—yet another unnatural substance that appears in produced milk—are often given.

Due to opposing viewpoints and the absence of long-term studies, parents have to decide for themselves. Adults who drink an occasional glass of milk need not be concerned, but when they have children who consume several glasses a day, parents may want to do some further investigation to help determine whether they will pay a little more and buy organic milk.

Chapter 14

Powerful Protein

Meat, poultry, fish, beans, nuts, seeds, eggs, soy, and dairy products are all rich in protein. Protein plays a very important role in building, repairing, and maintaining body tissues. It is especially needed during periods of rapid growth, as in childhood. Children should have two to three servings of protein daily to keep them healthy and growing adequately.

Limit the Red

Red meat, unlike plant foods, is high in fat and contains no fiber. For this reason, it moves more slowly through the stomach and intestines and can slow the elimination process.

Small amounts of lean red meat are a good source of protein, but frequent large portions over a period of time increase one's risk of obesity, cancer, and high cholesterol. **Red meat should be served in small portions a maximum of two or three times a week.** When considering serving sizes, red meat should be thought of as a side dish, not the main entrée.

Purchasing meat is a challenge, because so much of the selection is high in fat. Choosing the lowest fat varieties is advisable and, of course, these cuts are usually more expensive.

Prior to cooking red meat, all visible fat should be trimmed off. Red meat has a lot of excess fat marbled into it that cannot all be removed. Barbecuing or roasting meat will melt away some of this excess fat and allow it to drip off. Parents should avoid frying or baking in a pan where meat sits in its own juices, allowing excess grease to reabsorb.

To minimize meat intake, small amounts of meat can be diced up and put into healthy casseroles or added to stir-fried vegetables. With a variety of other tasty foods, small amounts of meat can be very enjoyable.

Pork, lamb, and veal are similar to beef in the amount of fat and calories they contain. These meats also should be eaten in moderation.

Fatty processed meats such as sausage, bacon, pepperoni, ham, and hot dogs should not be eaten on a regular basis. They contain a considerable amount of saturated fat and chemicals that are questionable for human consumption.

The First White Meat

Poultry is generally healthier than red meat. It is lower in calories and fat, and is easier for the body to digest. Unlike red meat, poultry does not have fat marbled within the meat. The fat is usually in clumps around the meat, so it can be easily removed.

Removing the poultry skin is advised to reduce fat and calories. This can be done before cooking if it will be cut up and added to soups, stews, or casseroles.

Skin can be left on while cooking when poultry is being baked, barbecued, or roasted. This keeps poultry from drying out. The skin then should be removed prior to eating.

White meat is the color of choice when it comes to poultry. It has significantly less fat and cholesterol, and fewer calories, than darker pieces do.

Chemical Contents

Organic meats of all types are preferable, but cost considerably more. Some livestock are given hormones and chemicals to make animals gain weight and remain free of infection. Unfortunately, consumers do not usually know what the meat they feed their families contains. It is a scary thought and a good reason to keep meat consumption—of all types—at a minimum.

Bushels of Beans

Protein can be obtained from sources other than meat products. Beans are among the more popular examples—they are also a great source of vitamins and minerals. Beans can be served warm or cold, and added to various main and side dishes. They also add nice color and texture to food.

Beans are naturally low in fat, but may have fats added to them during cooking or processing. Labels on canned beans should be read so varieties can be chosen that contain little or no added fat. Even refried beans can be purchased or made without fat. Beans can be eaten in small quantities, but also make a nice hearty meal for families with healthy appetites.

Nutty Nutrients

Nuts and seeds are little nutrient powerhouses. They are one of the best foods that can be eaten, because they are loaded with nutrients. Many adults shy away from nuts because they have a high fat content. What needs to be considered is that most of the oils they contain are the healthy type that are good for the heart and lower the bad type of cholesterol. Eating nuts may even prevent heart attacks.

Seeds are nutritionally similar to nuts. The reason for this is that seeds are nuts, just a smaller version. Nuts and seeds can be eaten alone, baked in breads, used in salads, and included in just about any dish. The rule of thumb for nuts and seeds is that a little goes a long way. They contain a lot of nutrients and a lot of calories, so a small amount provides the vitamins and minerals without excessive fat and calories.

Children under three years should not eat nuts. Due to their shapes and sizes, nuts may cause choking. Many children have also had serious allergic reactions to them. To reduce chances of harm or childhood death, parents should resist giving nuts to young children.

Sounds Fishy

Fish is protein-rich and full of vitamins. Substituting fish for meat is one of the healthiest dietary changes parents can make for their families. Unlike red meat and poultry, fish oil is actually beneficial to the body in modest amounts. Omega-3 fatty acids, found in some types of fish, actually help reduce bad cholesterol and increase good cholesterol. It also is good for cells in the brain, nervous system, eyes, and other organs.

Fresh fish may be steamed, baked, grilled, or pan-fried with nonstick spray. Frozen fish sticks and other fried fish are unhealthy and should be avoided. The breading and frying process undermines the nutritional value of any food. It makes no sense to take a perfectly healthy food and make it an unhealthy one by saturating it in harmful fats.

Canned fish packed in either oil or water is certainly an option. Fish packed in water is preferable, but fish packed in oil that is drained very well is acceptable as well. Fish is a nutrient-dense food that, if prepared in a healthful manner, is an exceptional choice for tasty, healthy meals.

Children of all ages can eat fish without difficulty, because it is easy to chew and swallow. Parents must cut it up into small pieces for children. Each small piece should be closely examined and all bones removed. Types of fish that have many small bones should not be offered to children at all—even with close attention to bone removal, a few may be missed. Fish without bones or with larger bones (easy to spot and remove) are a very healthy food choice for people of all ages.

Grade-A Goodness

Eggs are also a good source of protein. They are one of the highest quality sources of protein and very rich in vitamins and minerals. Egg white is essentially fat-free, cholesterol-free, and the most beneficial part of the egg. The yolk, however, does contain fat and cholesterol. For people who choose to reduce fat or cholesterol intake, eating a couple of eggs a week will not cause harm.

People who want to eat larger portions of eggs or eat them frequently during the week can do so by separating out and discarding some of the yolk. This way, a high-protein egg dish can be prepared with less fat and cholesterol. Eggs have received a bad reputation over the last several years, but in moderation they are a very healthy way to add protein to any diet.

Organic eggs are the best choice but are more expensive to buy. As with meat, consumers do not know how good the eggs they purchase really are. Chemicals given and diets fed to chickens vary greatly between farms. Some chickens are fed healthy feed, while others are fed garbage. Some chickens live healthy lives out in nature, while others live cooped up in pens and infrequently see daylight. All of these conditions reflect how nutritious eggs are. In general, eggs are a healthy food, but those people who have friends or family with a farm have a definite advantage.

Egg substitute is a great choice for an excellent-tasting high-protein food. Most brands are 99.9% real egg. They are cholesterol-free, fat-free, low-calorie, and contain many vitamins and minerals. They can be used for family meals and in place of eggs in recipes. Family members of all ages can enjoy tasty dishes made with this high-protein food.

Chapter 15

Sensational Soy

Soy is one of nature's most perfect foods. Gram for gram, no other food supplies as much nutrition as soy. It is high in protein, an excellent source of fiber, cholesterol-free, rich in vitamins and minerals, and supplies modest amounts of healthy unsaturated fats. Soy is a healthy alternative to less healthy, protein-rich foods like red meat.

Benefits Galore

Many Americans have just learned about soy and of its benefits. Other cultures have been eating soy for centuries. While American consumption averages only a few grams of hidden soy per day, various other countries consume averages of 50 to 80 grams per day. People in countries who eat a lot of soy live longer, have lower rates of cancer, and have lower incidence of heart disease.

The benefits of soy include:

♦ increasing bone density, therefore reducing the risk of osteoporosis
♦ reducing LDL (bad) cholesterol, while raising HDL (good) cholesterol
♦ reducing the risk of heart disease and cancer
♦ improving brain function

Tasty Tofu

Tofu is one of the most popular soy products. It is the curd of soybean protein. Unlike other products, tofu processing actually makes it more nutritious because its special processing increases the amount of calcium it contains.

Tofu can be purchased in a variety of types, depending on preference and use. All tofu is bland in taste, but nicely picks up flavors that surround it. Because of this, it can be added to different dishes for extra nutrition without changing the flavor of the original recipe.

Tofu can be served in many ways, including:

♦ adding it to stir-fry, soups, stews, sauces, or chili
♦ baking or sautéeing it in flavorful marinades
♦ pureeing it for dip, pate, or spreads
♦ blending it into fruit smoothies

Large amounts of oils are not needed when preparing tofu. Parents who are unfamiliar with cooking tofu can purchase a tofu cookbook to get them started. Versatility is a definite benefit of tofu, making it easy to fit into the daily diet.

Drink It Up

Soymilk is becoming more and more popular as people learn of the benefits of soy and incorporate it into their diets. Soymilk is made with nutrient-rich milk that is pressed out of presoaked soybeans.

Many brands of soymilk on the market are fortified with vitamins and minerals that increase the goodness of the drink. When comparing fortified soymilk labels to cow's-milk labels, parents can see that the nutritional facts appear very similar. While both beverages are exceptional sources of nutrients, soymilk is even better. Soymilk offers benefits that cow's milk does not, including:

- phytonutrients (reduce the risk of heart disease and cancer)
- less saturated fat
- less sodium
- no cholesterol or lactose

Although soymilk offers more health benefits than cow's milk does, children may enjoy consuming both on a daily basis. Having both on hand increases beverage variety.

Grocery stores stock soymilk on aisle shelves and in the refrigerator section. Flavors and consistencies vary widely from brand to brand. Some companies add extra flavor such as mixed fruit, vanilla, and chocolate which can also increase sugar content. Some brands are very flavorful and others are not. Families are advised to try several different types to find what suits them.

Take Your Pick

New products are frequently introduced that make soy an easy, healthy, and tasteful addition to the family diet. Readily available products include:

- roasted soybeans
- soy cheese
- soy pate
- soy coffee creamer
- soy eggnog
- soy yogurt
- soy dips and spreads
- soy hot dogs

Most of these items can be found in health food stores, and an increasing number of them are showing up on grocery store shelves.

Sacrifice the Sauce

Soy sauce should not be considered a healthy option for consuming soy. It contains excessive amounts of sodium and should only be used in minimal amounts. The low-sodium variety is better, but still has a high sodium content.

Overly salty foods are best not given to young children who are forming likes and dislikes. Children who get used to eating salty food may crave and eat too much salt for years to come. When parents are deciding which healthy soy products will be added to the family diet, soy sauce should be out of the running.

Greatness Prevails

Soy has cumulative affects, so the more years it is consumed the more benefit it has on the body. This is great for children who eat soy and continue to eat it throughout their lifetime.

Parents can add soy beverages very early in childhood. They can also begin feeding smashed or pureed tofu during the baby food stage. When children graduate into feeding themselves, parents can give them squares of baked or sautéed tofu. Firm tofu is very soft yet it holds its shape so it can easily be picked up and eaten—even without teeth.

Because of the naturally bland taste and odd consistency, many people claim their children will not eat tofu. When prepared well, it can become a family favorite. As with other attempts at pattern setting, it is beneficial to introduce tofu at an early age. If it is refused, further attempts can be made until a taste for it is acquired. Trying various recipes for tofu can be very helpful as well.

Fortunately, soy comes in a variety of products so chances are high that every family member can enjoy its marvelous benefits.

Chapter 16

Good Fats, Bad Fats

Dietary fats are an essential part of a healthful diet. Unfortunately, most Americans eat way too much of the wrong types of fat and too little of the beneficial types. This is a prime factor in weight gain as well as in many disease processes. To maintain a healthy diet and teach children to do the same, it is vital that adults have a basic understanding of good and bad fats.

Know the Limits

Recommendations for fat consumption vary depending on age. Children one year and younger require 40 to 50 percent of their daily calories from fat. They need the extra energy for rapid brain and body growth. Children and teenagers require less than 30 percent of their total daily calories from fat, and adults require less than 25 percent. Eating proper amounts of healthy dietary fat is very important, and equally important is consuming the right types.

Differentiating the Two

All dietary fats contain a mixture of saturated and unsaturated fats. The type of fat that predominates determines whether fats are solid or liquid, and characterized as saturated or unsaturated.

Fats such as lard and butter are solid at room temperature because they contain higher levels of saturated fat. Oils such as canola, corn, and soybean are liquid at room temperature because they contain higher levels of unsaturated fat. The degree of saturation is used to determine whether particular fats will help or harm the body.

Saturated Fat

Only a very small amount of saturated fat is necessary for healthy living and the human body naturally makes up what it needs. Unfortunately, Americans still consume quite a lot of it. Excessive amounts of saturated fat is incredibly harmful to the body and contributes to:

  ♦ weight gain and obesity
  ♦ high cholesterol
  ♦ organ and vascular system damage

When individuals do not minimize saturated fat consumption they develop plaque (fat build-up) along their inner artery walls. Over time plaque increases and little space is left for blood to flow through. Complete or partial blockage can occur. This leads to heart attack or stroke, either of which can be debilitating and life threatening.

Sources of saturated fat include:

 ◆ butter fat and lard

 ◆ tropical oils (coconut, palm)

 ◆ animal fats (meat fat, poultry fat and skin, and fat in whole-milk products)

Unsaturated Fat

Unlike saturated fat, unsaturated fat helps the body and is essential for a healthy diet. The vital functions of this good dietary fat include:

 ◆ aiding absorption and transportation of fat-soluble vitamins such as A, D, E, and K

 ◆ serving as an energy source

 ◆ building healthy cells and hormones

 ◆ building healthy brains, nerves, and other organs

 ◆ providing oils for healthier skin

Unsaturated fats can be broken down into two types—monounsaturated and polyunsaturated. The oils in each group are as follows:

Monounsaturated oils	Polyunsaturated oils	
olive oil	corn oil	flaxseed oil
canola oil	safflower oil	cottonseed oil
avocado oil	sunflower oil	grapeseed oil
peanut oil	soybean oil	sesame oil
	fish oil	walnut oil

When purchasing oils for home use, parents can keep in mind monounsaturated fats are generally healthier than polyunsaturated fats. Monounsaturated fats lower LDL (bad) cholesterol and raise HDL (good) cholesterol. Polyunsaturated fats, on the other hand, lower both types of cholesterol, which is less beneficial to the body.

Another advantage of monounsaturated oils is that they oxidize and turn rancid much slower than polyunsaturated oils do. If oils smell like paint or linseed oil, they have gone bad and must be disposed of. The shelf life of oils can be maximized by purchasing small bottles and keeping them tightly closed.

Unsaturated fats, especially monounsaturated, are an important part of maintaining good health, but one must still remember that too much of any type of fat is not a good thing. **All fats contain many calories and even the good oils contain some saturated fat. It is important to remember which oils are best, and that a little goes a long way.**

Consider the Sources

Some fats have been through chemical processing and may contain unhealthy additives that increase shelf life and make them less expensive to produce. These oils are "refined." Healthier oils can be located by spotting the term *unrefined* printed on the label. Obtaining unsaturated fats in their most-natural states is beneficial by far. Oils that are unrefined are not stocked at all grocery stores and may need to be purchased in health-food stores.

Oils found at health-food stores may be organic. This is an added benefit. Many oils that are not organic come from plants heavily sprayed with pesticides; therefore, pesticide residue remains in the oil. Organic oil is made from plants that are not sprayed with chemicals and is therefore better for the body.

Obtaining unsaturated fats can be done in a variety of ways. **It is advisable to eat nutrient-rich foods that naturally contain healthy oils in place of preparing food by adding fats of any type.** Foods like fish, avocados, wheat germ, nuts and seeds, and various nut butters provide other vital nutrients that oils alone do not provide. These foods are excellent sources of unsaturated fat, but as with all fats, they contain many calories and should be eaten in small amounts.

Adding fish to the family diet is definitely worthwhile, because it is very nutrient-dense and contains the healthiest of oils. These oils are called omega-3 fatty acids and are good for the heart and cholesterol levels. They may also reduce total fats in the blood, reduce LDL (bad) cholesterol, and raise HDL (good) cholesterol. The effects of these oils reduce the risk of heart attack and stroke by keeping blood products from clumping up in the bloodstream. Omega-3 fatty acids also improve brain function and body circulation. **It is recommended that at least one serving of fish high in omega-3, like salmon, trout, mackerel, tuna, herring, or sardines, be eaten each week.**

While cooking, it is worthwhile to consider how much and which oils are used in food preparation. **Deep-fat frying should always be avoided because this adds too much fat to the diet. Low-calorie spray should be used for most cooking.** Unsaturated fat then can be obtained from food itself and not from added oils. This will ensure that healthy foods are not made unhealthy by cooking in too much, or the wrong type of, oil.

Creating Havoc with Hydrogen

Hydrogenation is a process that uses hydrogen to change unsaturated fat to be structurally similar to saturated fat. This unnatural and unhealthy fat is referred to as hydrogenated fat, partially hydrogenated oil, trans fatty acid, and more commonly, trans fat.

Trans fat is as bad as, or worse than, saturated fat. Like saturated fat, trans fat raises LDL (bad) cholesterol and lowers HDL (good) cholesterol—this is a bad combination. **Trans fats are unnatural forms of saturated fat.**

The purpose of trans fat is to change the texture of oil from liquid to semi-solid form. Many food companies use trans fat instead of oil because it can reduce costs, extend storage life, and improve the flavor and texture of food.

Most processed foods eaten by children, including crackers, cookies, muffins, and peanut butter, contain trans fats. Parents serve foods such as these to children on a daily basis, therefore children are innocently consuming large quantities of foods that are harmful to them.

When health-conscious individuals want to know what particular foods contain, they refer to product labels. Unfortunately, trans fat is not listed on product labels as other fats are.

The FDA regulates what is put on the "Nutrition Facts" of food labels and unfortunately they have no current provision for including trans fats. As a result, most manufacturers do not offer such information to their customers. It is a scary thought that such harmful ingredients are present in so many foods without common knowledge of their existence.

Manufacturers are not only withholding vital information from consumers, but are adding insult to injury when they label processed foods with phrases like "no cholesterol" and "low in saturated fat" when they know the products contain resident trans fat that affects the body in the same negative ways as cholesterol and saturated fats.

To rectify this problem, because trans fat is proven to be extremely harmful to the body, the FDA is working on a new rule that will require trans fat labeling on packaged foods. Unfortunately, the new rule will not come into effect until January of 2006. Many large food-processing companies are actively researching ways to remove or reduce the amount of trans fat in their products, since they will soon be forced to openly display how unhealthy their foods really are.

Even though trans fat is not listed on Nutrition Facts labels, the approximate amount of trans fat in products can often be determined using a simple formula. The first step is to look at the listing of individual fats on a label. All of these fats (saturated, polyunsaturated, monounsaturated) are added together and deducted from the "total fat" amount. If partially hydrogenated oil or shortening is a main ingredient, it then can be assumed all or most of the fat remaining is trans fat.

For example:

Total fat:	12 grams
Polyunsaturated fat:	4 grams
Saturated fat:	2 gram
Monounsaturated fat:	1 gram

Add: 4 grams + 2 grams + 1 gram = 7 grams

Subtract: 12 grams - 7 grams = 5 grams

The 5 grams remaining are probably hydrogenated fats.

It is also helpful to remember that the closer to the top of the ingredient label trans fat is listed, the more the product contains.

To lower their family's intake of trans fat and saturated fat, parents can switch to reduced-fat, low-fat, fat-free, and trans-fat-free foods. It is also advised to switch to diet or whipped margarine and use it only in small amounts. These spreads contain less trans fat than tub and stick margarine. Products labeled "low in trans fat," or "contains no trans fat" can now be found in health-food stores and better supermarkets. These products are definitely worth purchasing and using in the home.

Most children love peanut butter. Since most brands contain a lot of trans fat, parents need to know how to choose those that do not. Peanut butters that contain trans fat do not separate while those that contain healthier fats do. If there is oil floating at the top of the jar, it is probably a good choice—to be sure, the ingredient labels should be read to confirm they do not list partially hydrogenated oil. The healthy peanut butters are typically called "natural peanut butter."

Unnaturally Unhealthy

The theory of imitation fats that contain no fat or calories sounds like a dream come true to many fat-conscious individuals—let us not be fooled. These products are fairly new on the market and long-term effects are still unknown.

Some people feel snack foods made with synthetic fat can be gobbled up with few or no negative effects, just because they are calorie and fat free. This is far from the truth. This "fake fat" is man-made and is not digested like natural foods are. In fact, it cannot be digested at all. The molecules that synthetic fat are made of are too large to be absorbed by the intestines. Because of this, the molecules never make it into the bloodstream, where fat and calories are utilized. Instead, the "fake fat" stays in the intestines, absorbing valuable nutrients and fat-soluble vitamins. The "fake fat," along with nutrients and vitamins, is then excreted as waste.

Synthetic fat causes uncomfortable side effects as well as lost nutrition. Amongst the most common side effects are abdominal cramping and diarrhea. A warning label is found in small print on the packaging of products containing synthetic fat.

When new man-made products come on the market, it is advisable to investigate them prior to consuming them. No surprises here—the best way to obtain the best nutrition is by consuming a variety of healthy foods in their most fresh and natural states.

Top It

When preparing foods, adding excessive amounts of butter or other unhealthy fats should be avoided. Flavor can be added with spices and foods like garlic and onion. When moisture is desired in drier foods like potatoes and pasta, topping with low-fat sour cream and low-fat sauces are great options. Stir-fried or freshly steamed vegetables also make great toppers for starchy foods. Parents can take advantage of low-fat and low-calorie sauces and toppings that add nutrition, instead of using those that add excessive fat and calories.

Food preference has a lot to do with pattern setting, so children who are served a healthy diet will have an excellent chance of preferring healthy foods throughout their lifetime.

Chapter 17

Sickening Sweets

Humans are born with a natural sweet tooth. This is shown by infant preference for sweeter fluids, such as breast milk, over those less sweet. Most foods, except those in the meat group, contain sugars of some sort.

The sweet tooth we are born with may be a genetic trait that exists to guarantee the body receives the energy it needs for survival. From an early age we learn to associate eating and drinking of sweet foods with pleasure. For these reasons it is not surprising many children, as well as adults, like sweets.

Sadly, Americans greatly over-consume sweets. Some people eat large amounts of them and do not think about or care about the consequences of such actions. Other people care about consequences, but find their cravings are stronger than their willpower. Others control their intake, but find it is a constant struggle. The fact is, people eat too many sweets, and the majority of the adult population would agree that avoiding sweets altogether is very difficult to nearly impossible.

Creating Cravings

Parents want to give their children things that bring them pleasure. A handy and inexpensive way of doing this is by giving them sweet treats. Unfortunately, if done frequently, parents are innocently doing their children a great disservice. They may be setting them up for a lifetime of sweet cravings, leading to unhealthy diets for years to come. Yes, we are born liking sweets, but giving the body excessive sweets can intensify the natural sweet tooth. This is why minimizing sweets in children is important.

Many lifetime patterns, good and bad, begin during childhood. Pattern setting should be a factor when determining how much, when, and which sweets will be allowed.

> **For example:** If a child is brought up eating sugary cereals every morning for breakfast, cookies or a candy bar every afternoon, dessert every night after dinner, or a big bowl of ice cream every night before bed, chances are the child will continue these or similar patterns into adulthood.

Many children at some point will be burdened with the battle of trying to fight "out of control" cravings and resisting patterns that have been ingrained. Instead of showing children pleasure through excessive sweets, parents can give them pleasure by providing them with excellent health and positive patterns they can carry on through the rest of their lives.

Other Options

Some parents limit their children's intake of sweets while others do not. Many parents feel a lot of foods like candy, cookies, and ice cream are all a big part of childhood and children might as well "enjoy them while they can." It is true that childhood should be a very fun time, but fun is not all about junk food. It is about things like a loving family, acting silly, playing tag, singing songs, and reading bedtime stories. Instead of giving children treats to keep them happy or quiet, parents can offer nutritious alternatives or engage in fun parent-child activities.

Problems Arise

People who excessively consume sugary food may crave it more frequently than others do. These individuals can substitute healthier snacks or simply cut down the frequency and amount of sweets consumed. In time, cravings may change so original foods are desired less and healthier foods are found to be more satisfying.

Sugars consumed affect the brain. Some people are more sensitive to sugar than others, and children generally are more sensitive than adults. When a balanced diet is maintained, the brain gets a steady supply of energy, and thought process is effective and consistent. On the contrary, when excessive amounts of sugary foods are consumed, attention span, learning, and behavior may be inconsistent.

Consuming excessive amounts of sugary food can keep the body from fighting illness efficiently. This can increase the number of illnesses acquired as well as lengthen the duration of each. On the other hand, when sugary foods are minimized and a balanced diet is consumed, the immune system is usually healthy and strong.

Consuming excessive amounts of sugary food will put fat on the body. This problem greatly contributes to the country's obesity epidemic. Because sweets have addicting qualities, and it takes a lot of them to make a person feel full and content, many people overindulge. These treats are very high in calories. Since the body does not need so many calories, it uses what it needs and stores the rest as fat. Those who continually overindulge, gain more and more body fat over time.

Sugar Incognito

Many families eat excessive amounts of sugar and do not realize it because foods contain hidden sugar. A few examples of these include:

- ♦ processed foods
- ♦ children's packaged foods
- ♦ canned food
- ♦ spaghetti sauce
- ♦ yogurt

Sugar may also be hiding in food under names not easily recognized as sugar sources such as:

- ♦ corn syrup
- ♦ dextrose
- ♦ fructose (natural sugar in fruit)
- ♦ glucose, glucose syrup
- ♦ honey
- ♦ invert sugar
- ♦ lactose (natural sugar in milk)
- ♦ maltose (natural sugar in grains)
- ♦ mannitol
- ♦ maple sugar
- ♦ molasses
- ♦ raw sugar
- ♦ sorbitol
- ♦ sucrose
- ♦ xylitol

A clue to remember is that words on an ingredient label ending in *ose* or *tol* may be sugar of some kind. Also, parents can be aware that labels claiming products are "sugarless," "sugar-free," or contain "no added sugar" may contain artificial or other sweeteners. Ingredient labels need to be read in order to determine what foods contain.

Many parents try to keep sugar out of their own diets, but allow their children to consume excessive amounts of it. Limiting sugar should be a family affair.

The only time sugary food should definitely be avoided is when children are under the age of one, and at any age when advised by a physician due to health issues. When children under the age of one are given sweets, it may interfere with their willingness to eat foods that are not sweet. Older children, however, could be allowed modest and infrequent sweet treats. Children who are totally deprived of sweets can become overly fascinated with them and that may create other problems over time.

When parents allow children their occasional sweets, they are best offered soon after a meal. This assures sugary treats are not replacing nutrient-rich foods. Having food in the stomach also prevents the blood-sugar fluctuations children may experience when sugary foods are eaten on an empty stomach.

It is advisable to keep only a couple of sweet foods and drinks in the house at one time. These items should be kept out of sight and reach of young children. As terrible as it sounds, hiding sweets from older children may be appropriate.

If parents feel the need to overindulge on sweets, they should do so when children are not around. This may seem unfair or cruel, but it is very important to set good examples.

Artificial Alternatives

Artificial sweeteners were originally used for people with diabetes, because they do not elevate blood sugar. Since they also contain few calories, and no sugar, marketers later directed their focus toward calorie-conscious people. The response has been phenomenal. Artificial sweeteners are now widespread and are added to thousands of different foods and beverages.

Food labels list sweeteners under various names, including:

♦ Aspartame

♦ Acesulfame Potassium (Acesulfame-K)

♦ Saccharin

♦ Sucralose

Artificial sweeteners are made of unnatural substances, and may affect the brain and body in unnatural ways. Consumption, especially by children, may cause harm and should not be taken lightly. Young brains and bodies develop very quickly and need the goodness of natural food to develop and thrive.

Another drawback of artificial sweeteners is they may not satisfy the body's craving for sweets. In fact, they get taste buds used to having excessively sweet food and drinks, so it may take more sweets to satisfy cravings.

Artificial sweeteners are still under investigation and long-term effects have not yet been determined. Because of this, frequent consumption may offer potential risks, so it is recommended they be consumed in moderation or avoided completely.

Pearly Whites

A very common problem of sugar consumption is tooth decay. Damage caused is permanent, but usually preventable. Cavities occur when food and plaque (an invisible scum) coat teeth. This coating changes to acid, eats the enamel away, and causes holes in teeth.

Before teeth can erupt, it is a good idea to wipe gums off daily with a wet cloth. As soon as the first tooth breaks through the gums, tooth brushing should begin. Early wiping and brushing keep gums and teeth clean, and get children slowly used to having oral care done for them. Starting early helps children better accept and tolerate the process.

When children get to the point of wanting to brush their own teeth, they can certainly take their turn, but until about seven years of age, parents must do a thorough job first. Allowing participation gives children practice in brushing as well as a feeling of pride and accomplishment of a job well done.

The best time to brush teeth is after meals and sticky snacks, before the food caught in teeth turns to acid. Until children are able to spit toothpaste out, parents should brush with a very small smear of regular or children's toothpaste.

Extra attention is required when brushing the teeth of children who have molars. Food gets stuck in ridges on top of the molars and can be missed. This is a common place for cavities to appear. **Parents must help with brushing instead of leaving it completely up to children who may not do an adequate job.**

It may be helpful to use electric or battery-operated spin toothbrushes for brushing children's teeth. The rotating bristles thoroughly clean with less manual circular and back and forth motion. They can be more expensive than regular toothbrushes, but are well worth the investment. Many children find spin toothbrushes fun and tolerate brushing more frequently and for longer periods of time.

Young children's teeth usually have spaces between them. If this is the case, flossing at a young age is not always necessary. Once children get molars or other teeth that touch, daily flossing should be started. Flossing is the only way to keep tight areas clean and cavity-free.

Dental checkups are recommended every six months, starting from age two or three. Good oral care is something all parents must provide and teach to their children.

Chapter 18

Halt the Salt

Sodium plays a vital part of regulating body fluids. The amount of salt needed to maintain healthy fluid balance is very minimal. The total amount needed is provided by foods in nature; therefore, it is unnecessary to add salt to anything.

Many packaged foods and snack items contain large amounts of added salt. Foods with added salt are fine every once in a while, but should not be consumed on a regular basis. Excessive salt has adverse effects on arteries and can increase blood pressure. This can create serious problems during adult years.

The majority of salt consumption comes from table salt, canned vegetables, processed meats, and snack foods. These should be limited. Table salt use can be reduced by removing salt shakers from cooking and eating areas. Salt consumption can also be reduced by rinsing canned vegetables prior to eating them. Processed meats contain chemical additives, preservatives, fats, and sugar, as well as added salt—there are much healthier sandwich-ingredient alternatives.

Snack foods contain different amounts of salt, so it is always advisable to read product labels carefully. To determine how much salt a food contains, the sodium column can be referred to. In most cases, lighter-salt snacks are preferable to those that contain more.

Children who become accustomed to eating salty foods will probably continue to eat them for the rest of their lives. When such children reach adulthood, serious health issues may arise. Individuals who incur such problems are usually advised to greatly reduce salt intake. By this point, damage to the vascular system has already occurred, and individuals find it very difficult to give salt up to prevent further damage.

People who do not consume excessive amounts of salt prevent long-term, salt-induced bodily damage. They also avoid the difficult process of attempting to reverse deeply ingrained negative patterns. As always, trying to change negative patterns is difficult, so it is best not to start them in the first place.

Chapter 19

Cholesterol Cautious

Cholesterol is fat that is transported through the bloodstream. It is found in foods like egg yolk, oil, and fat. A small amount of cholesterol helps the body and is necessary for normal body functions.

The amount of cholesterol and saturated fat consumed affects the level of cholesterol in the blood stream. When people overindulge in the wrong types of food, their cholesterol level can increase. Excess cholesterol in the bloodstream causes plaque to build up along artery walls. This process narrows the walls of the vascular system and constricts blood flow. **Significantly constricted blood flow is a serious condition with a high probability of causing heart failure or stroke.**

Lipoproteins are the vehicles that transport cholesterol through the bloodstream. High-density lipoprotein (HDL) is the "good" vehicle. It carries cholesterol from the arteries to the liver, where it is eliminated, thus lowering the risk of heart disease. A high level of HDL in the bloodstream is good for the body.

Low-density lipoprotein (LDL) is the "bad" vehicle. It carries cholesterol and deposits it along the inner walls of arteries, thereby contributing to heart disease. A high level of LDL in the blood stream is not good for the body.

HDL can be maximized and LDL minimized by consuming a balanced diet including moderate amounts of good oils and only very small amounts of saturated and trans fats.

Cholesterol is frequently spoken about in regard to adults, but plaque build up is a process that begins during childhood. Children who are active and consume healthy diets have a much lesser chance of having "high cholesterol" and excessive plaque buildup in teen and adult years than do those children who are sedentary and consume high-fat, high-cholesterol diets.

Positive habits are easier and healthier to start as children than to try to adopt as adults. Patterns to develop for a healthy heart and vascular system include eating foods low in fat and cholesterol, exercising regularly, and maintaining ideal body weight.

Chapter 20

Snacking Sensibly

Very young children have small stomachs, so they can only eat small amounts at any given time. Since they cannot eat enough to hold them over from meal to meal, snacks are vital for adequate nutrition. Older children have the stomach capacity to hold much larger amounts of food so they do not necessarily need snacks between meals.

Whether snacks are needed or not, most people eat several each day. Snacks can be very beneficial and be used to provide additional nutrition missed at mealtime. Unfortunately, many people eat snack foods containing excessive amounts of fat and sugar that provide few nutrients. Avoiding unhealthy snacks is as important as avoiding unhealthy foods at mealtime.

Because young children need to eat snacks between meals to satisfy hunger, parents can use snack times as additional opportunities to provide daily food requirements. When a variety of healthy, low-fat, low-sugar foods are served at snack time, limiting amount is not always necessary. Healthy and age-appropriate snack foods include:

- ◆ fruit
- ◆ melon
- ◆ vegetables
- ◆ whole-wheat bread or crackers
- ◆ cheese
- ◆ cottage cheese
- ◆ yogurt
- ◆ lean meat
- ◆ whole-wheat pasta
- ◆ finger sandwiches
- ◆ leftovers from prior meals

Older children often help themselves to snack foods as desired. When this is the case, it is still up to parents to monitor what types and amounts of snacks are being consumed. Otherwise, children may repeatedly overindulge in the wrong types of food. Parents will find it helpful to avoid keeping excessive amounts of junk foods in the home. This way, independent children will mostly have healthy foods to choose from.

Having healthy foods convenient and readily available increases chances children of all ages will eat them instead of less healthy foods. Usually when a snack is desired, we all want immediate gratification. Parents, as well as older children who can help themselves, will be more apt to choose healthy foods if little or no preparation is required. Quick snack ideas include keeping:

- ◆ a bowl of fruit washed and ready to eat
- ◆ a container of fresh vegetables washed, cut up, and in the refrigerator
- ◆ slices of cheese or lean meats available
- ◆ whole-wheat bread or crackers on hand
- ◆ a variety of healthy favorites like yogurt, cottage cheese, and no-added-sugar applesauce available

There are many snack foods parents choose with intentions of serving healthy foods, but in actuality some are not the best choices.

> **For example:** People hear the word "granola bar" and many immediately think "healthy." Granola is made of healthy grains, but often large amounts of sugar and oil are added (as in granola cereal) for flavor and consistency. To make soft granola bars, even more sugar and oil may be added. Some companies even increase fat and sugar content by adding ingredients like chocolate and marshmallows. When sweets are desired, granola bars are acceptable alternatives to candy bars, but they should not be considered healthy snacks for frequent consumption.

Reading labels before purchasing questionable snack items is highly advised.

There are many types of chips on the market and people of all ages find them irresistible. All chip consumption (except maybe those that are baked and lightly salted) should be limited. Nice alternatives to chips are whole-wheat crackers, low-salt pretzels, or crispy vegetables. These snacks can be enjoyed almost as much as chips—they are more nutritious and contain a fraction of the fat and calories.

Many adults and children snack out of boredom, anxiety, or habit. This can cause big problems for those who are overweight and for those who choose unhealthy snack foods. It is up to parents to make sure they have healthy foods available in the home, and their children are making smart snack choices, eating because they are hungry, and not spoiling their appetites for upcoming meals. When children eat for the wrong reasons, interventions need to take place. Physical and mental activities are great alternatives to unnecessary snacking for people of all ages.

Chapter 21

Drink Choices Do Matter

It is necessary to consume adequate amounts of fluid to maintain a healthy body. The very best beverage is water. Other excellent choices include low-fat milk, low-fat soymilk, diluted 100% fruit juice, diluted sports drinks, caffeine-free herbal tea, and low-salt vegetable drinks. These drinks supply nutrients without unhealthy additives.

Beverages to limit include soft drinks, juice drinks, juice cocktails, sweetened tea, punch, and beverages mixed from flavored powders that contain a lot of sugar. These drinks offer little or no vitamins and minerals. They also contain combinations of artificial colors and flavors, caffeine, carbonation, and large amounts of sugar or artificial sweeteners. When hydrating the body, it is best to give it only what it needs.

Soft-Drink Sabotage

Many parents choose to introduce soft drinks to infants and young children. This should not be done. Soda contains either artificial sweeteners or a lot of sugar (about 10 teaspoons per can), caffeine, and acid for carbonation. The caffeine can rob bones of calcium, sugar can rot teeth, and carbonation may upset young tummies. Soft drinks also have no nutritional value. Better options are drinks that provide vitamins and minerals, much less sugar, and no carbonation.

Most of the school-age children in this country drink soda, and about three quarters of them drink it every day. Adolescent girls average one a day, while boys of the same age average three a day. This amounts to hundreds of empty calories and large amounts of sugar or artificial sweetener each day.

Children who drink soda pop every day should be cut back to one or two per week or less. Other drink alternatives should be discussed with these children so both parents and children can agree on healthier options.

Juicy Misconceptions

Children today drink large amounts of fruit juice. Many parents are happy with this because they believe juice is nutritious. This is not completely true. It is acceptable to serve small amounts of 100% real fruit juice because it contains vitamins and minerals, but when juice is consumed in large amounts children get too much sugar and too many calories. Children are much better off eating a piece or two of fruit and drinking a glass of water or milk. This supplies vitamins, minerals, and a lot of fiber with less sugar than from drinking juice. Whole fruit is also much more filling than juice alone.

Many drink labels are made to fool customers into thinking products are real juice when they are not. Words like *drink* or *cocktail* usually mean "not real juice." These beverages are mostly sugar water with artificial coloring and flavoring.

Some may include synthetic vitamin additives or a small amount of juice. This allows labels to legally display phrases like "high in vitamin C" and "contains real juice." Parents should not be fooled—if a label does not say "100% real juice," chances are what is inside is not.

Real orange juice, not orange drink, is a good drink choice. It is full of vitamins and minerals and many contain no added sugar. Some orange juices are better than others.

Most orange juices have the water removed, then are reconstituted either at the factory (cartons) or in the home (frozen). These are fine choices, but may be slightly acidic and the flavor is frequently not that of fresh oranges. When purchasing this type of juice, the label should be read to make sure sugar is not added—oranges used for juice should be naturally sweet.

The best type of orange juice to buy are those that do not go through a reconstituting process. They are less acidic to the stomach and naturally rich in vitamins and minerals. They usually come in cartons and are found in the refrigerator section of most grocery stores. The labels read "100% pure orange juice," and "Not from concentrate." They taste just like fresh home-squeezed orange juice, and are often more healthy than concentrated versions are. These juices may cost a little extra but are definitely worth it.

Many children drink several glasses of fruit juice each day, which adds up to hundreds of extra daily calories. For this reason, all fruit juices should be diluted with at least 50 percent water. This cuts sugar and calorie intake in half and still provides nutrition, hydration, and a pleasant taste. If families establish only this new pattern, the rate of childhood obesity would drop. Drinking undiluted juices gets children too accustomed to sugary drinks, which makes water and other unsweetened drinks less palatable.

Diluting fruit juices rules out the convenience of children's juice boxes. Because they cannot be diluted, children get too much sugar and too many calories. Instead, colorful thermoses or sports bottles can be used. A little creativity can reduce sugar and calorie consumption, save money, and help our environment by reducing packaging waste.

Drinkable Vegetables

Vegetable juices can be made at home with a juicer or purchased at grocery or health-food stores. These are usually not popular drinks among children, probably because most parents do not think about them as options. Vegetable juices are very flavorful and definitely worth introducing, especially for children who do not eat enough vegetables. These juices do not have to be diluted because they are made of naturally low-calorie vegetables. As always, reading labels assures brands chosen do not contain added sugar or salt.

Most children, unless ill, have no problem keeping themselves hydrated. Children seem to love beverages of all kinds. Ideally, only healthy drinks are introduced during infancy and early childhood. Children who do not drink soda and full-strength juice will never miss it. Children who already consume these sugary beverages will need to be weaned off slowly.

Chapter 22

Organic or Not

Organic food is that which is grown in healthy soil with fertilizers that consist only of animal or plant matter. It is free of risky additives, including synthetic chemicals and pesticides. Foods that are truly organic are healthier, and eating them may decrease chances of bodily harm caused by eating foods that contain unnatural substances.

Purity Certification

Before October 2002, farming practices and standards were very unclear and it was difficult or impossible for organic consumers to know what they were purchasing. Labeling practices led consumers to believe they were getting something they really were not. After years of work, national organic standards have been implemented that should improve matters greatly.

Organic food producers and handlers now must be certified by a USDA-accredited certifying agent in order to sell, label, or represent their products as "100% organic," "organic," or "made with organic ingredients."

Small processors are certified only if they choose to be. Legally, smaller processors are exempt from certification but still must comply with applicable requirements if they wish to call their products *organic*. Only production or handling operations that meet certifying criteria may use the term *organic* on their labels.

Organic meat processing now has specific USDA standards that producers and processors must meet in order to label their agricultural products as organic. Edible livestock or livestock used for milk production must be managed on an organic operation in order to be sold, labeled, or represented as organically produced.

Chemical Accumulation

In modern agriculture, pesticides and other harsh chemicals are used. This leaves chemical residue on food we eat and in soil. There have been studies performed that confirm serious hazards of such chemicals, and we still do not know the extent of harm being done. Such hazards may become more apparent in a generation or two, when long-term effects arise.

Parents may choose to consider purchasing organic products for their children, whose developing bodies are especially susceptible to effects of toxic pesticides, fertilizers, and other chemicals. It is a precaution parents can take toward prevention of possible diseases in the future. Otherwise, unlike today's adults, children will consume these harsh chemicals for many, many years. Parents may not see effects of such chemicals in their lifetime, but our children or grandchildren may suffer the accumulative effects of them.

Reality Strikes

A problem with purchasing organic products is their cost may be considerably higher than that of nonorganic products. The reality is, many parents with young children are finance conscious and may feel they are unable to pay more than they have to for groceries. In these cases, parents may consider replacing just several regularly eaten products with those that are organic.

Some food items worth switching are:

- ♦ peanut butter and other nut butters
- ♦ nuts and seeds
- ♦ milk
- ♦ cooking oil
- ♦ 100% fruit jams
- ♦ meats

The nonorganic versions of these particular products may contain larger amounts of chemicals than many other foods. By giving up products that carry health risks for those that do not, parents may actually be saving money in the long run by saving on future medical expenses occurring from eating contaminated food for long periods of time. Above all, serving children food that is uncontaminated gives parents the satisfaction of knowing they are not doing their children harm by feeding them chemicals or pesticides.

Health-food stores are wonderful for picking up organic products, whole-grain and whole-wheat products, healthy bulk foods, and specialty items, but when it comes to other shopping, cost-conscious consumers may want to shop around. Some items can be purchased while on sale, or for less money at grocery stores. As with anything else, it pays to compare products and prices.

Organic products are often more expensive because they cost more to produce. The plants and animals are given high-quality, chemical-free nourishment and are raised on chemical-free farms. These practices are very costly to maintain. Because pesticides are not used, organic farms do not always produce blemish-free, marketable products, so there is a waste factor as well. The results, however, are that plants and animals raised under such conditions are void of unnatural substances, packed full of vitamins and minerals, and usually taste great.

Many fruits and vegetables that are not organic can be reduced of chemical residues prior to eating. Much of chemical residue resides on the outer surface of fruits and vegetables. Foods with skins like bananas, oranges, and kiwi are the easiest—they just need to be peeled prior to eating. Foods that do not require peeling, like apples, tomatoes, and lettuce, should be washed well prior to eating.

Some residues are oil based so washing with water alone may not be enough. A dab of dish soap diluted in water can be used. Parents who choose not to buy organic produce can minimize chemicals consumed by their families just by peeling and washing foods.

Chapter 23

Television Trends

Watching television promotes inactivity and consumption of large amounts of junk food. Such a combination is a definite setup for weight gain and disease.

Minimizing Modern Technology

For a fun time, children used to run and play. Now they sit in front of computers and televisions. Not only are the children content with this lifestyle, but many parents are too. One of the problems of computers and television is they often replace physical activity. **The more time people spend on computers and watching television, the less time they spend exercising the body.** Parents can ensure a healthy balance if they insist children take part in a moderate amount of active work or play each day. Children may be surprised being active can be even more fun than watching television or playing video games.

Television not only encourages inactivity, it encourages consumption of large amounts of high-calorie, high-fat, and high-sugar foods. While concentrating on television programs, people often consume large amounts of snack foods. Some people are used to eating when they watch television so even if they are not hungry, they grab something to snack on anyway. A good way to avoid consumption of extra calories is to make a family rule that all food must be eaten in the kitchen and away from the television. This will make every family member more aware of eating habits and reduce needless snacking.

Televisions should not be on during mealtimes. Many children overeat while watching television because their appetite control signals are ignored. Some children undereat while watching television because for them the distraction displaces attention away from food. Some of the best conversations can take place at mealtime. Parents can encourage positive family interaction and positive eating patterns by leaving the television off.

Targeting Children

Television advertising affects children's eating habits, without a doubt. The food industry takes full advantage of this and directs marketing to children. Children see commercials and ask their parents to buy the products advertised, and many do. This amounts to billions of dollars in revenue for companies selling fast food, soda pop, sweets, sugary cereals, and other foods children would be better off without. American children are exposed to about ten such food commercials per hour of viewing. Commercials teach children food should be fun rather than a source of nutrition. To reduce exposure to such big-business marketing schemes, parents need to monitor viewing and help choose the stations their children watch.

Limiting Exposure

Even when appropriate programs are selected, there is no reason why children should spend more than one or two hours a day watching television. **Children's viewing time must be limited.**

Parents who decide not to expose their children to television programing at all have other entertainment options. There are excellent videos that can be rented, purchased, or checked out from libraries. In many cases, videos are better than television. They are commercial free, may teach children various age-appropriate skills, and end after a period of time and can then be shut off.

Because videos have a definite start and finish, setting limits is often easier than with television that has ongoing programming and commercials. Another good point about videos is, even when in another room, parents know what their children are being, or not being, exposed to.

Teaching the Truth

Delaying exposure to junk food marketing schemes for as long as possible is advisable, but sooner or later, exposure will occur. At this time, it is advisable parents teach their children to be skeptical about advertising.

Children can learn they should not believe everything they see on television or any other mode of advertising. The older children are, the better the chances will be they will accept and understand this reasoning.

When older children ask for junk food they have seen advertised on television, parents can read and discuss food labels with them. These are great opportunities for educated explanations of why certain foods may not be acceptable choices. This approach should be better tolerated than just saying "no." Parents may then choose to assist their children in comparing labels to find healthy alternatives children and parents are happy with.

Chapter 24

Forego Fast Food

There are hundreds of thousands of fast-food establishments in the United States, and American fast-food consumption has increased five-fold in the last twenty years. These trends are driven by enormous advertising and marketing campaigns, and by the consumer's desire for fast meals at minimal cost. Because fast food is inexpensive and readily available, parents frequently choose it over preparing healthier meals at home.

Quantity over Quality

New technology allows the food industry to produce a huge variety of processed and packaged foods and beverages. This enables fast-food giants to provide much of what the world eats. Much of the food supply fast-food industries demand is very inexpensive and greatly overproduced, so they can afford to sell large meals for small prices.

If fast-food customers are looking for quantity, they are getting a great deal, but if they are looking for quality, they are getting a rotten deal. Fast foods tend to be low in fiber, vitamins, and minerals, and high in trans fat, saturated fat, and sugar. These are the components that cause obesity as well as increase risk for various other diseases.

Prioritizing Meal Preparation

These days, families seem to be busier than ever, and parents often find themselves too busy or too tired to cook for their families. Meal planning and preparation does take time and effort, but if it is made a priority it can be done without too much difficulty.

Preparing healthy meals for their families is one of the most important things parents can do. Years of eating healthy foods compared to years of eating unhealthy foods can mean the difference between a long, healthy life and a shorter, less healthy life. Few things in life are as important as good nutrition and children deserve nothing less.

Family meals do not have to take hours to prepare or be made fresh every day. When a meal is being prepared, it takes little extra time, effort, or mess to make a double or triple batch. Leftovers can be frozen or refrigerated for future snacks and meals.

Some parents may choose to cook several meals all at once, in preparation for the whole week. Come mealtime, it is very convenient to choose the meal, heat, and serve. It is very rewarding for parents to know they are feeding their children good wholesome food without heavy cooking every day.

Indulging Intelligently

There may be times, whether away from home or in a hurry, when fast food seems like the only option. It is fine to indulge, as long as it is not on a regular basis. When ordering fast food, choices can be made to add nutrition and reduce trans fat, saturated fat, sugar, and calories. Options include:

- ♦ skipping mayonnaise and special sauces; ordering mustard, ketchup, pickles, onion, or hot sauce instead
- ♦ skipping fries and chips; asking for extra vegetables instead
- ♦ avoiding cheese and double meat
- ♦ avoiding sour cream and butter
- ♦ requesting whole-wheat bread
- ♦ ordering water or low-fat milk instead of soda

It is best not to purchase actual child's meals. They offer foods with little nutrition that are very high-fat. **One child's meal can provide calories for a whole day with just a fraction of the recommended daily nutrients**. When children eat fast food, as with any food, it is up to their parents to make the healthiest choices possible.

Made-to-order sandwich shops are a great alternative for more healthy fast food. Many of these establishments offer whole-wheat bread and a large variety of fresh vegetables and low-fat meats. When sacrificing the cheese, mayonnaise, and oil, and skipping the chips and soda, these sandwiches make tasty meals that are healthy, filling, and low in fat.

Parental Planning

Frequently, parents know ahead of time when families will not be able to return home for meals. On these days, parents can pack healthy meals or snacks. This will save the family from eating whatever is close and convenient—especially since close and convenient may be unhealthy and expensive.

When food is prepared ahead of time, persons preparing the food are usually not yet hungry. This allows them to carefully plan and prepare nutritious meals without hunger getting in the way—at mealtime the food is ready to eat. When healthy foods are readily available, family members are less likely to grab quick, unhealthy foods out of pure hunger. For the small amount of time and effort it takes to prepare food to go, families receive a lot of benefit.

The Dirty Truth

Some fast-food industries target children, as well as adults, to deliberately "hook" them on their food. After all, if they succeed they have customers for life. Such actions are definitely not in the best interest of people at any age.

Lawsuits have been filed against some fast-food restaurants because certain individuals feel they have suffered great bodily harm from consuming large amounts of fast-food. Some people believe fast-food packaging should contain warning labels to advise consumers of what they are eating, but only a few restaurant owners provide such labeling. Some individuals claim fast food is not only unhealthy, but addictive.

While all of this may or may not be true, the facts are the food is fast, convenient, and unhealthy. Unfortunately, too many people consume too much fast food and many have become very unhealthy and overweight because of it.

Most adults know that fast food is not a healthy choice, and whether they eat it or not is a decision they make. Most children, however, do not have the knowledge or understanding to make the same educated choice. They know what tastes good, what their friends are eating, and what offers the most fun (at least as advertised).

Infrequent meals at fast-food restaurants may be acceptable, but parents need to be cautious that negative life-long patterns are not initiated by those visits. It is up to parents to decide when, what, and if fast food is appropriate for their families.

Chapter 25

Restaurant Reality

Families who eat healthy the majority of the time can surely eat out at restaurants now and then. Parents definitely deserve an occasional break from meal preparation and cleanup. There are many ways families can enjoy the benefits of eating out and still receive fairly healthy meals.

By Special Request

Menus usually give a brief description of what food is served and how it is prepared. Parents can use this information to decide which dishes are the healthiest choices and choose from those.

It is important to remember that food prepared by others is very likely to include hidden fat, salt, sugar, and chemicals. Customers, unfortunately, have no idea which or how much of these substances are added. If in doubt as to how a food is prepared, it is wise to ask prior to ordering.

Restaurants put effort into making food as tasty as possible, but few put effort into making food healthy, as well. When ordering, parents should not hesitate to ask for what they want. Special requests may include serving:

- ♦ butter, oil, salad dressing, fatty sauces, and gravy on the side
- ♦ whole-wheat bread instead of white
- ♦ salad or unbuttered, steamed vegetables instead of fries, chips, and creamed soups

There is no reason to eat unhealthy food just because restaurant personnel choose to serve it this way. It pays off to let needs be known by people who are expected to meet them. Customer satisfaction is a primary goal for restaurant staff. After all, this is how they earn their pay and keep customers coming back for more.

Indulging Intentionally

Amounts served in restaurants may be considerably more than families eat at home. This can add hundreds of excess calories to meals. Parents should not feel that any family member must eat excessive amounts to get their money's worth. Extra food can be packaged up, taken home, and served as another meal or snack a day or two later. When eating out, as when eating at home, it is important that adults and children listen to their bodies' natural signals and stop eating when they have had enough.

Discipline or Disaster

Salad bars and all-you-can-eat buffets are great for some people and disastrous for others. It all depends on individual preference and discipline. People who like fruits and vegetables and stop eating when they are full may be happier making their own individual food selections and determining amounts. On the other hand, people who are unable to resist eating large amounts of high-calorie, high-fat prepared salads and foods are usually better off ordering a meal instead. Because salad bars and buffets offer a variety of healthy and unhealthy foods, it is important that parents know which fall into each category so appropriate choices can be made.

When eating at salad bars and buffets, best choices include:

- ◆ fresh vegetables
- ◆ fresh fruits and melons
- ◆ beans
- ◆ seeds
- ◆ nuts
- ◆ whole-wheat breads
- ◆ unprocessed lean meats
- ◆ low-fat, frozen yogurt (if dessert is desired)

Salad-dressing application should be kept to a minimum, and low-calorie versions are usually the best choices. Serving salad dressing in a separate bowl can help prevent over-usage.

The worst commonly chosen foods from buffet style restaurants are:

- ◆ potato and pasta dishes that contain large amounts of mayonnaise or oil
- ◆ anything fried
- ◆ heavily buttered vegetables
- ◆ mashed potatoes and gravy
- ◆ macaroni and cheese
- ◆ chips
- ◆ creamed soups
- ◆ pizza
- ◆ buttered white bread
- ◆ muffins and sweet breads
- ◆ desserts

The list continues, differing from restaurant to restaurant. Just by looking, it is usually easy to differentiate between healthy foods and unhealthy foods. Unless advised differently, it can be assumed mayonnaise used in restaurants is not the low-fat variety and oils used are not the healthiest types. Healthier versions of these products do not always come in the less-expensive economy sizes restaurants purchase. Salads can be prepared at home using choice ingredients, but when prepared in restaurants this is not usually the case. **When eating at salad bars and buffets all family members should eat larger quantities of healthy foods and much less of the unhealthy foods.**

Appetizing Temptations

Appetizers in restaurants are usually unhealthy and should be avoided or kept to a minimum. Most appetizers on menus are breaded and deep-fried. Those that are complimentary are usually fried chips, white bread and butter, or other unhealthy snack foods that cost restaurants very little money to serve.

Unfortunately, appetizers are very tempting because they are placed on tables when customers are hungry and anxiously awaiting their food. People who are disciplined, and do not have children who will fixate on the snack foods, may accept appetizers and eat only a very small amount. This is difficult for most people to do.

Even foods that otherwise would be avoided may not be resisted when they are placed on the table of a hungry family—the best option is to decline such foods altogether. Even when such foods are complimentary, families that refuse them are not missing out on anything but extra fat and calories.

If appetizers are desired, parents are better off ordering clear soups, salads, or fresh vegetables. Parents with young children can even bring age-appropriate fruits or vegetables for children to eat while waiting for meals to be prepared. The fruits and vegetables will not spoil appetites and can prevent hungry children from becoming overly fussy. Offering such foods is an excellent way to take advantage of the hunger and undivided attention of children to increase the amount of healthy foods they consume.

Drinking Excess Calories

Drink options in restaurants are often high in sugar and can add many unnecessary calories to meals. Children who drink soda and other sugary drinks frequently fill up on these fluids and take in less food. This increases sugar and calorie consumption while decreasing nutrient intake.

Ordering water or low-fat milk instead of sugary beverages is highly advised. Children then will not overindulge in sugar, and are likely to take in more nutrient-dense food. Parents with children who drink instead of eat may choose to limit all fluids prior to and during meals. This will increase the appetite for food.

Dining out requires planning, with careful consideration given to ordering healthy foods that can be enjoyed by all. It is definitely worth remembering that when fewer unhealthy foods are taken in, more healthy foods will be consumed in their place. The opposite is unfortunately true as well. By making appropriate food and beverage choices, parents can assure proper nutrition for every member of the family.

Chapter 26

Realistic Remedies

The trick to avoiding unhealthy foods is having the knowledge and ability to prepare meals that are healthy. When time is short, even parents who are well advised in family nutrition become tempted to serve unhealthy foods that are quick and easy. Now and then, such meals are fine. In fact, it is not realistic for parents to serve a perfectly balanced diet all day, every day. Anything can be eaten on occasion, but the large majority of meals and snacks should be healthy.

Most parents should have little difficulty understanding the facts presented in this book. The hardest part is actually incorporating them into a busy family life. Below is a list of healthy foods that can be easily prepared. These and many other foods that require cooking need little to no added oil or butter—nonstick pans and cooking spray work great. Spices and low-fat condiments can be added as desired.

Any of the following foods can be changed to meet family preferences, and several foods can be combined to make meals complete. Experimenting with foods and preparation techniques can greatly increase variety and improve nutrition. Following are some examples of the many nutritious, quick foods that can be prepared. Parents with young children must be cautious to choose and prepare only those foods that are age-appropriate.

Lunch and Dinner Foods

- baked or grilled fish
- burritos made with whole beans or fat-free refried beans, whole-wheat tortillas, and vegetables of choice
- whole-wheat pasta with spaghetti sauce
- chicken, turkey, or vegetarian sandwiches on whole-grain bread or bagel with vegetables of choice
- chicken fingers made by cutting chicken breasts into fingers and baking or sautéeing (great for sandwiches, salads, or dipping in low-fat dressing or honey mustard sauce)
- lean hamburgers or garden burgers served on whole-wheat buns with vegetables of choice
- soy hot dogs wrapped in whole-wheat tortilla or bread
- chicken and vegetables of choice, wrapped in whole-wheat tortilla
- steamed vegetables sprinkled with Parmesan cheese
- cold vegetables with fat-free dip (either raw or previously steamed)

- pasta salad made with steamed or raw vegetables, black olives, apples, nuts, and a small amount of healthy oil or dressing of choice
- potato salad made with nonfat mayonnaise
- child's salad with mixture of favorite vegetables, beans, beets, fruit, olives, nuts and seeds—mix in a small amount of low-fat dressing or cottage cheese
- cottage cheese mixed with yogurt, fruit, or applesauce
- fajitas with lean beef or chicken and vegetables of choice; serve on corn or whole-wheat tortilla with low-fat sour cream
- baked potatoes topped with low-fat sour cream and steamed vegetables
- mashed potatoes made with low-fat sour cream instead of butter (great with garlic, too)
- baked, broiled, or barbequed lean beef or chicken
- stir-fry vegetables (can add lean beef, chicken, seafood, or tofu)
- rotisserie chicken purchased from a grocery store (remove skin and fat)
- baked chicken (remove skin and fat after cooking)
- brown rice cooked in low-fat, low-sodium chicken or vegetable broth
- whole beans and brown rice
- humus or tofu pate on whole-wheat pita bread with vegetables of choice
- tuna salad, turkey salad, or chicken salad made with nonfat mayonnaise, diced apples, onion, and celery
- steamed vegetables covered with low-fat pasta sauce
- brown rice topped with steamed vegetables of choice
- baked or boiled fresh yams
- fresh, frozen, or canned vegetables
- whole turkey (takes hours to cook, but nice for leftovers)
- baked or sautéed tofu
- enchiladas made with chicken or lean beef, onion, and a small amount of cheese (warm tortillas in microwave instead of frying)

Snacks

- whole-wheat crackers and a small amount of cheese or natural peanut butter
- rice cakes with nut butter of choice
- homemade, low-salt popcorn, popped with minimal oil (microwave popcorn is high in trans fat)
- vegetables alone or with low-fat dip
- bananas, carrots, celery, or apples with natural peanut butter
- fresh or dried fruit
- cottage cheese

Desserts

- fresh fruit
- yogurt
- low-fat ice cream or frozen yogurt
- sherbet or sorbet
- popsicles
- whole-wheat graham crackers
- cottage cheese topped with fresh fruit
- applesauce
- raisins or other dried fruit

Drinks

- water
- nonfat or low-fat milk (whole milk if between the ages of one and two)
- low-fat soymilk
- diluted 100% fruit juice
- undiluted vegetable juice
- diluted sports drinks
- caffeine-free, herbal tea (warm or iced)
- warm, diluted apple cider

Chapter 27

Consistency with Care

At a very young age, children learn how to trust from parents who consistently come when they cry, feed them when they are hungry, and change their diapers when they are wet or soiled. In a very short time, children unconsciously notice the repetition and therefore learn about cause and effect. These are beginning stages of childhood pattern setting.

Positively Positive

Positive and negative patterns are set in a similar fashion, and they occur whether parents realize it or not. Parents that are aware of this and utilize positive pattern-setting strategies have a definite advantage over those who do not. These parents frequently have better-behaved children as well.

> **For example:** Children frequently ask for things like candy and are told "no." If parents are consistent and hold firm to their "no" answer, even with persistent children who ask again and again, the children learn that "no" means "no" and they quit asking. These children learn their parents mean what they say and it is not helpful to keep harping about it. However, if parents are not consistent and sometimes give in to children who keep asking, children learn they can get what they want if they are persistent in bothering their parents. These children also learn not to take their parents at their word on future issues.

A Joint Effort

It is helpful when parents and other caregivers have a similar approach to pattern setting and together maintain consistency. Children then learn that what one person says or does is not drastically different from another.

> **For example:** When both parents insist that their young children always eat a nutritious breakfast, the children do not know any differently and do just that. If at some point one or both parents start allowing sugary sweet cereal or doughnuts for breakfast, consistency is broken. The children will begin wanting junk food in the morning and may refuse nutritious breakfast foods previously enjoyed.

Patterns help children learn what to expect. Using consistency to establish positive patterns allows children to grow up to become confident, trusting, and healthy adults.

Difficult but Determined

Raising children is not easy. It becomes even more difficult when parents are busy, tired, or both. When children are crabby on top of it all, parental frustration can set in. These are times when it is most difficult to be consistent.

Tired, overwhelmed parents may let consistency slide now and then out of pure exhaustion. Reminding themselves of the importance of consistency may help parents dredge up the energy needed to do what is necessary during these times.

When parents let consistency slide, children are usually the first to notice. Children then either become confused or realize they can get away with something they could not get away with before. After patterns are broken, parents have to work extra hard to reestablish them.

Areas of pattern-setting may include eating, house rules, chores, sleeping, or any other area desired. When setting patterns of any type, consistency is a must.

Chapter 28

Positive Parenting Patterns

Parents shape their children's behavior in all aspects of life, including dietary patterns. An ideal family situation includes parents who eat adequate amounts of a variety of healthy foods. After all, what children see at home is normal for them and in their eyes it is how it is supposed to be. When parents teach food discipline, they must set good examples.

Like Parents, Like Child

In order for children to develop positive eating patterns, parents must display such patterns. Children see parents as role models. If parents tell children one thing and do another, children become confused.

> **For example:** Some parents drink soda pop at dinner, but serve milk to their children. When children ask for soda instead of milk, parents may respond by telling children they do not need soda because it is not good for them. This is unfair and confusing to children. They wonder why it is alright for their parents, but not for them. The parents in this example would be better off drinking what their children are allowed to drink and saving tempting soda for times when they are away from their children.

In order to set good examples, it is vital that parents "practice what they preach." Positive examples should be set, not only with types of food and beverages consumed, but with amounts as well. If children see parents frequently overindulging, chances are their children will do the same. This is one reason why many overweight parents have overweight children.

Bad eating patterns that some parents possess are not always those of overeating. Some parents undereat or maintain overly strict diets. Children with role models such as these have a greater chance of developing eating disorders like anorexia nervosa or bulimia.

Do as You Say

Many parents believe in the phrase "do as I say, not as I do," and enforce rules accordingly.

> **For example:** Parents may have coffee and cookies for breakfast but insist their children have oatmeal. This is a double standard that will cause problems in the future. Children may obey parents to avoid punishment or flat-out refuse to eat the oatmeal. Either way, the children become confused and do not truly believe the reasoning they are told.

Children are smart and know when something just does not seem right. This can cause a lack of trust to develop. In a situation like this, children may rebel when given the opportunity.

To help parents further understand how their behaviors affect their children, they can place themselves into their children's shoes. Parents can ask themselves how they would feel if they were experiencing the double standard. Realizing how important positive role models are to children may help parents fulfill these roles to the best of their ability.

Role Model 101

Becoming a positive role model takes work and does not happen overnight. To get started, parents can make a list of several patterns they would like to initiate. Beside each entry, steps can be listed that will be taken to develop and solidify the pattern. Each person involved must have a clear understanding of the goal and of their duties.

> **For example:** A family who wants to give up eating decadent desserts after dinner each night can do so by writing down "minimize desserts" as a goal. Steps then can be listed of what it will take to achieve this goal. Steps may include serving fruit, yogurt, or applesauce when sweets are desired, playing a game or going for a family walk after dinner, not frequently buying or preparing rich desserts, and designating one day a week when a rich dessert will be allowed.

Young children do not need to be directly involved in the process of establishing patterns. They will learn indirectly by new patterns family members display.

Children who have positive role models can grow up with a more secure foundation, as well as a deep feeling of trust and respect for their parents.

Chapter 29

Pleasant Persuasion

Children generally tolerate mealtime and eat more nutritiously when parents are neither overbearing nor overpermissive. When parents sway too far in one direction or the other, complications may arise.

Getting children to eat certain foods can seem impossible at times. Parents often become frustrated and use hostility and pressure tactics to get children to eat foods they reject. Unfortunately, forcing the issue does more harm than good. It frequently results in confrontation between parents and children, ending with children resisting foods more adamantly than ever before. Parents usually find pressuring children to eat does not work.

Forgo the Force

Instead of forcing children to eat certain foods, some parents swing to the opposite side of the pendulum. They let their children have whatever they want to eat in order to keep peace and avoid upsetting the children. This is a terrible pattern to get into for the following reasons:

- ♦ It teaches children they have the ultimate say in what they eat and do not eat.
- ♦ Children are less likely to develop a taste for a variety of foods and they may not get proper nutrition.
- ♦ Children are more likely to develop weight problems and other health issues.

It is up to parents to provide a variety of healthy foods for their children and it is up to children to decide whether to eat what is being served or not eat at all. Parents, of course, should make sure they serve one or two foods they know their children will enjoy with each meal. Children who are very stubborn may miss a meal or two if they want to eat different foods. It will not take them long; however, to learn that if they are hungry, they eat what is being served or they undergo the discomfort of an empty stomach.

Try and Try Again

Like adults, children have foods they love to eat and those they do not. While children should be encouraged to try new foods, they should not be forced to eat foods they truly do not like. Such actions may cause them to refuse trying new foods in the future.

Small amounts of disliked foods should be served now and then, and children should be encouraged to taste them. The foods may be ignored or pushed off the plate for a period of time, but after about eight or ten samplings of a particular food, children are likely to develop a taste for it. When children are given frequent opportunities to try new foods, they are more likely to develop a wider range of tastes.

Children that are curious about food are frequently willing to try different types. Such curiosity should be encouraged. Comments advising them they will not like particular foods should be avoided—even when foods had been disliked in the past. Children should be able to make up their own minds about what they like and do not like and be able to change their minds over time. Most parents will agree, there are already enough foods children claim to not like without adding more.

Children should be allowed to try just about any food. Warnings should be given when appropriate, as with spicy foods, so there are no surprises that promote fears in trying new foods. In cases when particular foods are not appropriate for children, as with those containing alcohol, honest and age-appropriate reasoning is advisable. In most circumstances, when children show interest in new or previously disliked foods, it is very beneficial to offer them a taste.

Using Food Foolishly

Withholding food as punishment should not be done: for example, taking food away for using bad manners or spilling milk at dinner. This increases the value placed on food and can cause children to become preoccupied with food. With children of all ages, verbal correction or punishment is necessary at times. Appropriate options for discipline include time-out sessions or removed privileges that do not involve food.

Offering nutritious foods in a relaxed, nonpressured atmosphere is the best way to get children to maintain a healthy diet. Since children learn by example, parents should take part in mealtime rituals. Children can be taught that eating nutritious meals with loved ones can be an enjoyable experience.

Chapter 30

Receiving Rewards

Eating patterns could very well be set up by psychological factors that begin as early as hours after birth. Children learn that eating relieves discomfort as well as provides feelings of pleasure, comfort, and security. As children grow older they continue relating food with these positive feelings.

Promoting Problems

Many parents unknowingly abuse the natural association between food and pleasure. They offer foods, usually sweets like candy and cookies, to reinforce desired behaviors. Rewarding with food creates exaggerated food associations and undesirable eating patterns.

When food is used for rewards during childhood, it is likely it will also be used for rewards during adolescent and adult years. Individuals who reward themselves with food may also use food to deal with uncomfortable feelings such as boredom, hostility, sadness, and depression. Using food to feed emotions can cause serious issues with health and weight control.

Outstanding Options

Nonfood rewards are useful to people of all ages. Items like stickers for young children and allowances for older children teach the value of working and deserving something for a job well done. Showing children how to earn what they want is a great tool for teaching them one aspect of adult life.

Although rewards can be beneficial, children should not receive tangible rewards for everything they do well. Rewards can be solely the positive feeling that comes with accomplishment and praise.

The most recommended reward for children is verbal praise. This creates a loving feeling for both parents and children. Hugs or pats on the back can intensify feelings experienced by both parties. Life should be full of pleasant rewards. It is when they revolve around food that problems can arise.

Older children and adults who have learned to use food as reward and comfort measure end up taking in many more calories than they otherwise would. Food choices at such times are usually high in fat, sugar, or both. This not only increases junk food consumption, but it fills the stomach and therefore decreases healthy food consumption. This is how many people become unhealthy and overweight.

Once patterns are created, they can be very difficult or impossible to change. For some people, the inability to change such patterns can create a lifetime of misery. Ideally, positive eating patterns are set up at a very early age, allowing energy and emotions to be used on the happier aspects of life.

Chapter 31

While in the Care of Others

Many children are taken care of by day-care providers, babysitters, nannies, relatives, or other qualified caregivers at times during their lives. While in the care of such individuals, patterns are set and reinforced just as they are when children are with their parents. It is important that parents advise caregivers of rules and limits to enforce regarding nutrition and activity.

Here, There, and Everywhere

Many children in the country today are in day care full-time. This means children may eat more meals away from parents than they do with them. In these cases, it is vital that caregivers have a clear understanding of the eating patterns parents wish to instill and maintain.

If caregivers are providing meals and snacks, parents should know what they consist of and how much is allowed. If food served does not meet parental expectation, parents may request that changes be made. Parents also may choose to bring their own food for their children. In many day-care centers, "brown-bagging" is a requirement. It works great, since children have likes and dislikes, and parents can prepare foods they want their children to eat. Eating arrangements and foods served is an important point to inquire about when evaluating and arranging child care.

Win, Win Situation

When caregivers are being paid to do a job, there are expectations from all parties. When expectations are met, everyone is happy and the working relationship continues. When loved ones care for children, especially when not paid, the rules may change.

Grandparents, relatives, and friends who are especially attached to children may want to show love by serving special foods or offering excessive treats. This can become a problem. Parents often do not feel comfortable expressing that they are displeased with such actions. It is very helpful when limits and expectations are verbalized ahead of time—then friendly reminders can be added as needed.

If loved ones insist on giving treats, parents can request they be either nutritional snacks or nonfood items like puzzles or books. Parents may find it helpful to tell loving friends and family members that the children are fond of them regardless of treats and gifts they provide. Most people who take care of children want to do what is best for them—they just may need a little educating and gentle guidance on what exactly is best.

Exercise Expectations

When children are with caregivers on a regular basis, physical activities should be a consideration. Parents can choose not to allow children to watch TV, play computer games, or sit around excessively. Caregivers are working, and keeping children entertained is part of their job.

Caregivers may plan their own activities that provide exercise for children, as well as activities that stimulate thinking. Other caregivers may not be as imaginative and require more direction. For these individuals, parents can leave lists of games and activities caregivers and children can do together. A basket filled with toys and games left for babysitters may be helpful. Activity can be fun, promote health, burn calories, and promote bonding for closer relationships.

Eating nutritiously and maintaining active lifestyles are big steps toward living happy, healthy lives. For this to occur, parents may find it helpful to involve anyone who plays a significant role in raising their children. Caregivers can establish positive or negative patterns in children, so it is up to parents to make sure the patterns being established in their absence are ones they approve of.

Chapter 32

Finding Balance

Because obesity has become so common, more people are realizing they may be at risk. People of both sexes, all weight categories, and all ages are aware of waistline differences between individuals.

Many children as well as adults are so concerned about being or becoming overweight, they take extreme measures to lose weight or keep from gaining it in the first place. Instead of maintaining adequate weight with proper nutrition and exercise, more and more people are seeking drastic measures that are harmful and sometimes deadly.

Educational Enlightenment

Children become aware of weight differences as early as preschool. Along with awareness can come worry of becoming overweight. At or before this point, it is helpful for children to be educated about healthy eating and exercise.

Children should be taught that thin does not always mean healthy. Children who appear infatuated with models in magazines and catalogs should be told of the extreme dieting, surgery, and airbrushing of photos frequently involved with producing such pictures.

It may be helpful to explain that all bodies are unique and that it is impossible for most people to look like many of today's models and be healthy, too. The many benefits of a strong and healthy body and mind should also be discussed.

Problem Intervention

Families react differently to children who overeat and gain weight or undereat to lose weight. Some children become so out of control with food issues, even the best family intervention does not help. Other children come from families that are oblivious to such problems and do not realize anything unusual is occurring. Some families are aware of problems, but either do not take them seriously or do not know what to do. Such situations are very unfortunate.

Children obsessed with eating may become obese and those obsessed with weight loss may become anorexic or bulimic. Eating disorders (overeating or undereating) can occur in early childhood. Parents with children of all ages must begin steps of prevention if problems are suspected. Interestingly enough, similar steps of prevention can be used for any of these problems even though some, like compulsive eating and starvation, are opposite in nature.

Parental Pattern Improvement

The prevention of unhealthy pattern setting in children involves role models, since children watch parents and learn from what they do and do not do. Parents have many legitimate excuses, like working long hours and maintaining high stress levels, but the truth is that many are extremely poor role models when it comes to eating.

Parental eating habits range from excessive to inadequate. Both may involve unhealthy food choices, frequent talk about the need for weight loss, and sometimes even the use of diet pills, diet drinks, and laxatives—all of which can be hazardous to one's health. Most people are somewhere between the two extremes, but in most circumstances there is room for improvement.

Adults who have fallen into negative eating habits may find them difficult to change. For some, being healthier and having healthy children is enough of an incentive to improve their patterns. Others choose not to change their own patterns at all. When this is the case, parents should not talk about weight concerns or display unhealthy patterns around their children. With any luck, this may prevent the passing of bad habits on to children.

Parents who eat adequate amounts of healthy foods, limit junk food consumption, and avoid displaying extreme dietary habits are most likely to raise children with healthy eating patterns.

Creating Self-Image

Children who have, or think they have, developed a weight problem are likely to develop low self-esteem. The problem may be intensified by peer pressure, which includes a desire to be attractive and popular. Resulting anxiety may drive children in one of two ways: One, they turn to food for comfort. This usually causes weight gain, more feelings of inadequacy, more anxiety, and even more weight gain. Two, they turn the opposite direction and refuse to eat adequately. This can result in serious weight loss and illness.

By assisting to create a positive self-image in their children, parents may be able to help prevent low self-esteem from occurring. This can be accomplished by teaching children nobody is perfect and by offering praise about positive attributes their children possess.

Compliments should be genuine and can be on anything, including special abilities, talents, strengths, or outer beauty. Compliments and praise can create a positive self-esteem and help prevent children from becoming insecure, and vulnerable, and from developing a distorted body image.

Keep It to Yourself

While positive comments toward children are greatly beneficial, derogatory remarks about anyone can be harmful to children who may be listening. Children pay careful attention and put a lot of thought into what they hear.

When children are repeatedly exposed to negative comments, they begin to believe a person's body appearance is overly important. This may be all that is needed for them to start having unhealthy thoughts about weight. Avoiding such comments in the presence of children can prevent them from fixating on weight issues. It can also prevent children from developing prejudices.

If the topic of weight loss comes up, it is helpful to make only constructive comments to children.

> **For example:** Discussions with children regarding their need for weight loss can be addressed in a positive manner. By focusing on the need for children to become healthier, their feelings are less likely to be hurt and a healthier mind-set will be established.

Developing strong concerns about obtaining the ideal figure can become problematic for children, while developing strong concerns about obtaining ideal health is greatly beneficial.

A Happy Medium

Parents are usually the first to notice when their children are eating inadequately. Whether they are continually eating too much, too little, or making bad food choices in general, parents frequently are inclined to intervene. Stepping in is often necessary, but parents must be very cautious on how they handle situations, so they do not make matters worse.

Children who eat too much and are becoming overweight should not be overly restricted on the amount of food they are allowed to consume. Those who are overly restricted frequently become determined to eat as much as they want. They may frequently feel unsatisfied and begin sneaking food. Food may become overly important to them and they may fixate on it. This sets them up for patterns of overeating for years to come.

Instead of restricting food, parents can change amounts of types of foods served. Serving sizes of high-fat, high-calorie foods can be smaller, while serving sizes of low-fat, low-calorie foods can be larger. Foods such as salads, vegetables, whole-wheat bread, brown rice, and fruit can be offered to fill them up. This way they do not leave the table hungry and thinking about more food.

Children who eat too little should not be forced to eat. Those who are forced may refuse food even more. They also may become resentful toward parents who are doing the forcing. This is why it is helpful to serve appropriate foods and let children decide how much they will eat. Chances are, when children do not eat their meals they will certainly be hungry for the next one and can make up lost calories then. Light, nutritious snacks can be offered between meals, but they should not be substantial enough to spoil the appetite for the next meal.

Ideally, children consume adequate amounts of nutritious foods and refrain from eating excessive amounts of junk food. With very good intentions, some parents strive for perfection and put children on overly strict diets—this is not beneficial. Completely eliminating unhealthy foods from the diets of children does not work and can harm future eating habits.

Children who are raised on very strict diets may feel resentful toward parents and alienated from peers for being different. When these children are older, they frequently sneak prohibited foods. Parents cannot completely keep children from eating junk food. **The trick is to teach children about moderation.**

Chapter 33

Dangerous Disorders

The number of people becoming overweight has been dramatically increasing. At the same time, people are becoming more preoccupied with slenderness. Many children and young adults are taking drastic measures to become thin, risking their health and lives in the process. For many, becoming thin is an obsession.

Diseases Defined

Anorexia nervosa is a disorder characterized by severe weight loss without known physical illness. Young people with this disorder have an intense fear of becoming obese. The fear does not diminish as weight loss occurs. Sufferers claim to feel fat even when emaciated.

Without treatment, people with anorexia nervosa refuse to eat enough to maintain a healthy body weight. Refusal to eat is usually triggered by personal crisis or traumatic interpersonal incidents. Weight loss seems more and more important until it becomes out of control. Frequent triggers include teasing, the growth phase of puberty, and family stress. A commonality is sufferers feel they have no personal control. These people find the decision to eat or not is an area they can completely control.

Bulimia is a disorder characterized by binge eating. As with anorexia nervosa, young people with this disorder have an intense fear of becoming obese. Sufferers of bulimia eat large amounts of high-calorie foods over a short period of time, then purge by self-induced vomiting or diuretic and laxative abuse. Rigorous exercise is also sometimes used to burn absorbed calories.

Bulimic individuals are frequently depressed and have been unsuccessful at dieting in the past. They have difficulty controlling their impulses and often were self-conscious about being overweight at a young age.

Complex Commonality

Although eating disorders can occur in both sexes, they most commonly occur in females. It is most frequently seen in young people between the ages of 12 and 21.

Although frequency is increasing, an exact cause has not been identified. It appears to be a complex equation that involves a combination of internal factors and outside influences. Some young people definitely appear to be more susceptible than others. Those who are more susceptible are greatly influenced by thinness promoted through television, movies, magazines, and catalogs. Such outside influences become unrealistic role models for young people.

Room for Improvement

Parents who are overly concerned with their own weight and are frequent dieters or overeaters need to take extra precaution with their children. Such parents may become so preoccupied with their own food and weight issues they forget about teaching their children to eat healthy and promoting normal growth. Dieters and overeaters often try to establish healthy patterns within their children, but find they are unsure of normal food regulation. This is because many overeaters and chronic dieters actually forget or have never been taught how to eat normally.

When people adapt eating patterns, whether positive or negative, they often stick to them and fail to consider other dietary habits as possible options. Adapting unhealthy eating patterns from parents can be hazardous for children as they may become overweight or malnourished, fail to develop properly, become prone to illness and disease, or develop eating disorders of their own. These children start off life with one strike against them.

Adults with bad eating patterns may or may not choose to make changes for their own sake, but as parents they should attempt to do what is best for their children. The process of improving dietary habits can be gradual. Small steps toward positive change can amount to miles of benefits.

Home life is a significant factor that, unlike others, parents have some control over. Developing healthy eating patterns early in life and having good role models may prevent eating disorders. If eating disorders occur, in spite of a parent's teaching efforts, knowledge and positive patterns learned during childhood can be very useful during recovery. By establishing good eating habits in children, parents have nothing to lose and everything to gain.

Parents can do their best, and still not be able to prevent eating disorders in children. Unlike obesity, early stages of anorexia and bulimia are difficult to detect. Many sufferers realize others would not approve, so they keep eating patterns secret and hide their thinning bodies by wearing baggy clothing. Parents who suspect their children are eating too much or too little should contact their child's physician without delay.

Chapter 34

Exercise Is for Everyone

In America, one out of every four children is overweight and numbers are increasing. Healthy eating habits and increased physical activity are needed to transform today's society of unfit and overweight people into a society of healthy people. Maintaining balance between calorie intake and expenditure is exactly what is needed to achieve and maintain this goal.

Since the country is experiencing an obesity epidemic, it is obvious Americans are consuming too many calories and expending too little energy. Individuals of all ages who are overweight should focus on eating appropriate amounts of a variety of nutrient-rich foods and increasing physical activity.

Active Advantages

Years ago, most people led physically active lifestyles, but in the age of computer technology this is no longer the case. We now have to find ways to incorporate exercise into our lives. Many people know they should exercise, but still choose not to. Exercise must be a priority in life or it will not be done. It is unfortunate so many people are sedentary, because the benefits of exercise are so great. Some of these benefits are:

◆ reducing the risk of many diseases like high blood pressure, diabetes, and heart disease

◆ slowing the aging process and helping body systems to function more efficiently, which reduces stress and increases life span

◆ burning calories, increasing body metabolism, and temporarily suppressing hunger

◆ increasing muscle mass, adding body tone, and increasing strength

◆ boosting immunity, lowering cholesterol, reducing the risk of cancer, improving digestion, and building a healthy heart

◆ building stamina, increasing coordination, lubricating joints, and providing energy

◆ minimizing mood swings, improving concentration, and building self-confidence

Physical activity can be started at a very young age. Activities like reading, coloring, and listening to music are very important for childhood development, but so is exercise. **To become healthy and well-rounded individuals, children need both mental and physical stimulation.**

Encouraging Movement

Exercise for young children is usually very simple to initiate. In early childhood, exercise is just active play. Self-motivated children or those with siblings or friends of similar ages may not need encouragement. On the contrary, some children are not self-motivated and do not have other children to play with. Some children prefer low-stimulation activities above more active ones. In such cases, parents can facilitate active play.

Great Fun

Exercise for young children can be done without special gadgets or high-tech machinery. Many children use imaginary play and make up their own games, while others require a bit of direction and teaching. Simple activities like jumping rope, dancing, running races, and riding bikes, skateboards, or scooters provide exercise. Other physically active games can be taught to and played with children including:

- ◆ Hide and Seek
- ◆ Tag
- ◆ Ring-Around-the-Rosy
- ◆ Leap Frog
- ◆ Duck, Duck, Goose
- ◆ Hop Scotch
- ◆ Simon Says

Children who have developed a moderate amount of coordination may enjoy playing sports at an early age. Child-friendly sports include gymnastics, basketball, kickball, softball, swimming, and racquet sports. Activities can be modified so they are age-appropriate for young children.

If equipment such as ropes, baseball bats, and racquets are necessary for activities, parental supervision and guidance is necessary. Teaching children to swim and ride bicycles at an early age is also appropriate. With activity in mind, parents and children can use their imaginations to make up their own activities.

Creating Programs

As children grow older, free time for activity often dwindles. Between school, after-school activities, computers, television, and homework, many children become sedentary. During this time they discover school vending machines and cafeteria food that frequently results in unhealthy food consumption.

School-aged children who are involved in sports like swimming or track, which require sustained vigorous activity, have an advantage over those who are not. Their choice of exercise works their muscles as well as their cardiovascular system. Those who are involved in anaerobic sports, like weightlifting, work their muscles well, but work their cardiovascular system to a much lesser degree. These individuals can greatly benefit from incorporating aerobic exercise into their regimen.

Sadly, many school-aged children are not involved in sports or other exercise programs. Even though children's lives are very busy during school-aged years, time must still be made for exercise.

Exercise, like people, comes in many shapes and forms. Young people might want to select several types they may enjoy—or can at least tolerate. Having more than one exercise option keeps boredom from setting in and burnout from taking place. Variety allows young people to make choices, and this gives them a feeling of control and independence.

Staying with It

Starting and sticking with an exercise program is one of the hardest parts of exercise. People find many reasons and excuses why they do not exercise. Such people need to make excercise a priority, decide on an actual program, and commit to it.

Once the commitment has been made, it is helpful to find ways to guarantee it is fulfilled. Exercise appointments can be written down in appointment books or on calendars. This guarantees days are not filled up with other commitments, leaving no time for exercise. Exercise dates can also be set up with reliable exercise partners several times a week. This makes exercise more fun, and partners can support and help each other maintain goals.

People also can attend set classes on certain days every week. This creates a specific pattern and other engagements are planned around the classes. Attending the same classes each week becomes less intimidating for shy or insecure individuals because exercise routines and people become familiar. What works for one person may not work for another, so the trick is to find what works best on an individual basis.

Indoors or Out

Some people prefer exercising outdoors while others would rather be indoors. Brisk walking and running are especially nice for people who like to get outside. They are exceptional choices for burning calories and require no special skills.

People who prefer to be inside can attend exercise classes or use exercise videos. These options are beneficial because they offer instruction on proper technique as well as motivation. Many video stores and libraries carry a wide variety of exercise videos that can be taken home and viewed. This is a great way to make choices before purchasing videos for home use.

Regardless of indoor or outdoor preferences, everyone should have several options for exercise they enjoy doing. Individuals who do not do the same routine over and over will be more likely to enjoy exercise and less likely to get bored and quit.

Getting Serious

Health clubs and fitness centers are great for people who become motivated when surrounded by weights and fancy machinery. Young people who find they fit into this group may choose to join an exercise facility.

When joining, new members should always request an equipment demonstration. Anyone who uses exercise equipment should fully understand how equipment works, how it can be adjusted for individual body size, and which machines work which muscles. They also need to be instructed on the use of proper body mechanics to obtain maximum benefit and remain injury-free.

Exercise facilities usually offer a variety of classes as well as specially trained staff to assist members with establishing appropriate routines according to personal goals and abilities.

Memberships to exercise facilities can be quite costly. When several family members are interested in joining, family memberships can usually be purchased at a reduced rate. Children who are very motivated to workout in such facilities who cannot afford fees may have other options to obtain membership.

Many facilities offer memberships in exchange for a couple of hours of work each week. This can be very beneficial. Children not only get a membership free or at a reduced rate, but have the opportunity to learn about fitness from more experienced employees and members. To inquire about co-op programs, parents can contact exercise facilities in their area. Most exercise facilities are great places for older children to get exercise as well as develop a circle of friends who are interested in health and fitness.

Goal Establishment

When younger children play games like tag, they are acquiring cardiovascular benefit without realizing it. It is a shame we outgrow childish games that are so beneficial to our health. Health-oriented older children and adults replace fun childish activities with regimented exercise programs. Just about everyone would agree exercise may not be as fun as playing tag, but nonetheless can be enjoyable and above all, it is a necessity for healthy living.

Prior to starting any exercise program, individuals should obtain their physician's approval. Once this is done, individuals may choose to seek information and guidance from professionals in the exercise field. Bodies are different and react differently to exercise so monitoring is advised.

Every workout must begin with at least a five-minute warm-up and a light stretching period. Then children can start their chosen activity at a moderate pace and slowly increase duration and intensity over a period of time. Twenty minutes is an adequate cardiovascular workout goal for healthy children beginning an exercise program. During this time, children should be breathing hard, but not so hard they are unable to hold a conversation. The routine should always end with a cool-down period of at least five minutes and more stretching. Stretching after a cardiovascular workout is most beneficial since muscles are more elastic when they are warm.

Aerobic exercise should be done a minimum of three to four times a week. Exercise may seem difficult at first, especially for out-of-shape and overweight children. Over time, exercise will become easier as bodies become more conditioned to activity and excess weight is lost. Without a doubt, the benefits of exercise are well worth the effort.

Everyone, including enthusiastic older children, must start exercising very slowly. A common error is doing too much, too soon. This makes the body very sore, overly tired, and prone to injury. Exercise should not feel unbearable. Starting slowly and gradually increasing duration and intensity is very important. Small changes in activity level burn extra calories and prevent excessive discomfort and harm.

Choosing a Lifestyle

Exercise does not always have to be structured. Family activities are a great way for families to spend time together, have fun, and get some exercise. Ideas include:

- going on hikes or nature walks
- riding bikes
- skating, skate boarding, or roller blading
- swimming
- dancing
- exercising to videos
- playing outdoor games

At times when house or yard work is a priority, children may be able to lend a hand by doing age-appropriate chores. Cleaning may not be much fun but, aside from helping their parents out, it keeps children moving and prevents them from sitting around and snacking. Offering children choices of several different jobs or activities may be helpful.

Young people who take part in planning their own activities have a greater chance of sticking to a plan. No matter which activities are preferred, it is very important children get into the habit of maintaining an active lifestyle.

In addition to exercise routines, young people can burn calories and further increase metabolism by incorporating short episodes of activity into daily life. Ideas include:

- riding bikes or walking to nearby places instead of riding in cars or buses
- climbing stairs instead of taking elevators
- playing outside or going for walks instead of watching television
- washing family cars instead of playing computer games

Basically anything that replaces sedentary entertainment with calorie-burning activity is beneficial.

An active lifestyle not only benefits the body physically, it provides a psychological boost as well. Active people spend less time sitting around feeling sorry for themselves, and less frequently consume extra food out of boredom or depression. People who do aerobic exercise produce increased levels of chemicals that create a euphoric feeling. These chemicals, called endorphins, are good for the body and help keep exercisers committed and coming back for more. No matter what the preferred exercises are, most people receive a nice mental lift from activity in general.

Family Affair

Parents who exercise regularly have a better chance of raising active children. Even parents with very young children can exercise. Strollers and baby joggers allow parents to speed-walk or jog for exercise, while young children enjoy the view. Toddlers and preschoolers can get exercise by walking the last couple of blocks while parents slow their pace to cool down their bodies. Stopping at a nearby park or playground is also a nice opportunity for children to burn off some energy and reward them for good behavior during exercise time.

To make outdoor activity with young children more convenient, parents may choose to keep a bag of necessities packed that are needed during outings. Of course, items will change according to season. Ideas include:

- diapering supplies
- sunscreen, sunglasses, and shade hat
- rain gear
- cool-weather clothing
- water
- nutritious snacks
- blanket
- toys
- cell phone for emergency use

Parents who exercise with small children will most definitely find outings much less stressful if they do not have to gather all necessities every time they go out. The easier and more enjoyable exercise is, especially with young children, the more willing parents are to do it regularly.

When packing for exercise outings, snacks should be nutritious. Children use association in their everyday lives, and if they receive sweet treats once or twice during exercise outings, they will expect them and may even demand them each time. It is nice when children learn to enjoy the adventure and not ignore it while focusing on goodies.

Parents with preschool or young school-aged children can maintain speed-walking or jogging programs while their children ride bikes, skateboards, scooters, or roller blade alongside them. This way everyone gets some exercise and has fun, too.

Safety First

Wherever there is information about exercise, safety must be mentioned. Exercisers of all ages should drink plenty of fluids (preferably water or diluted sports drinks) before, during, and after exercise to avoid dehydration. Appropriate clothing should be worn for activities. Shoes do not need to be top-of-the-line, but should fit properly and provide adequate support and cushioning.

Protective equipment like helmets, goggles, and padding should be worn when engaging in activities where injuries are more likely to occur. Sports and exercise equipment can be quite costly. Parents may choose to purchase used equipment or less-expensive brands to be used in beginning stages. Parents also can keep in mind sports clothing and gear make great presents for gift-giving holidays.

Parents need to be aware of potential problems associated with some types of childhood sports and physical activities. Sports like gymnastics, wrestling, and ballet may mandate unhealthy weight control. Many coaches encourage, and may expect, performance that ultimately could jeopardize a child's health. Drastic weight loss and weight gain in such children has been known to cause permanent health issues. When children are required to reach or maintain certain weights in unhealthy ways, parents and their children need to seriously consider finding other sports or sources of exercise.

Moderation Is Key

Females, as well as males, who are overly active need exercise, health, and weight monitoring to assure they do not overdo it. Exercising obsessively or participating in various high-energy sports can cause athletes to become very thin. In some cases weight loss is intentional and in some cases it is not. Either way, excessively low body fat in females can cause hormonal changes that stop menstruation. This is a sign they may be overtraining, undereating, or both.

Excessive eating and exercise behaviors that go on for a significant period of time can cause serious irreversible physical and mental damage. Parents who suspect such behaviors should seek medical attention as soon as possible.

In the athletic environment, school-aged children—mostly boys—may come in contact with people selling steroids. People can make steroids sound very impressive but do not mention the long list of terrible side effects steroids cause, including organ failure and death. Some school-aged boys and young men become overanxious to develop quickly and build large amounts of muscle mass— steroids may sound like a quick way for them to get this wish.

Children need to be taught that excellent health and a strong, healthy physique are obtainable purely through good nutrition and exercise. Children who are very driven can push themselves hard to achieve realistic goals as long as they have proper instruction and supervision. Exercise is beneficial, but can be harmful if health and safety are disregarded.

Chapter 35

It's Never Too Early

Fat babies are not necessarily healthy babies. Although many grow out of their chubbiness, some do not. Ninety-nine percent of infantile obesity has no physical cause, therefore proper diet and activity would prevent most cases. Many overweight babies are raised with overweight parents, siblings, grandparents, or caregivers. In many cases, these individuals are not ideal role models and do not set adequate limits for children. Despite the cause of weight gain, steps can be taken to decrease chances of children becoming overweight adults.

In a perfect world, all healthy babies would be raised with patterns written about in this book. If this was the case, the obesity epidemic would not exist and disease, anxiety, and depression would be greatly reduced. People would live longer, and millions of overweight people would be thinner, happier, and healthier. Unfortunately, this is not a perfect world.

Predicting Patterns

Allowing or promoting undesirable behaviors lays the foundation for potentially harmful lifetime patterns.

> **For example:** Some parents feed their babies every time they become fussy. Unless parents suspect their babies are hungry, it is desirable to cuddle or play with them, change their surroundings, or change their diapers. Crying does not always mean babies are hungry, and feeding them every time they cry sets up patterns of using food for comfort.
>
> Allowing babies to carry a bottle around with them sets up a similar nonproductive pattern.

Patterns like these seem harmless during early stages, but they increase risk of eating for comfort in later years. Eating for comfort and snacking all day can lead to weight gain and health problems.

During the first year, babies eat large amounts because they are developing and growing very quickly. Normally, this allows them to triple their birth weights within this time period. Although they take in a great deal of calories, it is important to remember that their stomachs are only about the size of their fists. This allows them to eat only small amounts at a time, and since small amounts of food do not last long, they need frequent feedings.

Toddlers grow taller while weight gain slows and they usually slim down as they begin walking and become more active. Their eating habits often reflect such changes. It is perfectly normal for toddlers to continue eating large amounts, eat moderate amounts, or become nibblers.

Each body requirement is different, and children who are allowed to listen to their bodies will eat their required amount of calories. Young children usually let parents know when they are hungry. It is the job of parents to watch and listen for such cues and provide healthy foods when cues are given.

During the first couple of years of life, children listen to their bodies much more than older children and adults do. Such awareness should be encouraged. Unless babies are underweight, parents should resist the temptation to continue feeding babies who pull away from a bottle, breast, or spoon of food. Pulling away or refusing to open their mouths is a clear sign they are no longer hungry. Forcing the issue by trying to get them to finish a bottle of formula or expressed breast milk or a jar of baby food teaches babies they should override their internal, natural feelings of fullness. Ignoring such feelings can become an ingrained pattern of behavior that may continue throughout life.

Diet Modification

During the first few years of life, children grow very rapidly. During this time, attempts should not be made to reduce weight. Instead, parents of overweight children can try to slow down the rate of gain by providing healthy foods and limiting those with high calories and little nutritional value. Fruits, vegetables, low-fat milk products, and whole-grain products can replace more caloric foods. Overweight children in this age group who are active and consume a healthy diet will usually grow into their weight without excessive food restrictions.

During the toddler and preschool stages, children tend to eat slowly and the amount of food consumed each day may fluctuate drastically. This is normal and healthy. Eating slowly but steadily should be encouraged. Some children may need pleasant reminding to eat while others may not. Expecting or allowing children to eat very quickly should be avoided. People who eat quickly often consume many more calories than those who eat slowly, and many fast eaters find themselves overfull after meals.

Many parents are concerned about their young children not getting enough nutrition so they insist their children eat everything on their plate. Such actions are not encouraged. This frequently causes unnecessary disputes between parents and children. It also creates negative feelings for children in regard to meals that can create some food-related anxieties. Forcing children to eat all of the food on their plate teaches them to ignore their biological intake mechanism and patterns of overeating can be set.

While parents choose the foods that are to be served, children should be allowed to decide how much they want to eat. The exception is in cases where children tend to frequently overeat. In such cases, parents may choose to serve an adequate amount of food and give seconds if desired. When children ask for more, it is appropriate to say "no" and remind them that when their stomach is no longer hungry it is time to stop eating. They can be reminded if they overeat they may get a stomachache. It is helpful to tell children they can have more food at snack time, the next meal, tomorrow, or whenever is appropriate. This may alleviate feeling they need to eat a lot because they may not get any more food.

Early Education

The toddler and preschool years are the formative years for development. This is when children learn to make food choices and understand how food is supposed to make them feel. These years are very important for forming lifetime dietary habits. Parents can take advantage of their influence during these years and begin teaching about good nutrition.

Communication is very important during early school-aged years. Simple explanations like "these foods make you grow tall and strong and those foods do not" may be sufficient. Children with increased intelligence require more in-depth explanations of what and why changes are taking place. Children often eat healthier foods when they are given choices.

> **For example:** A parent may say to a child, "I've fixed you a whole-wheat tuna sandwich with fat-free mayonnaise and carrot sticks for your lunch, instead of having you buy a hamburger and fries at school. This is a more healthy lunch with much less fat. Would you like to take a bottle of sports drink with you, or do you want to buy a carton of milk at school?"

Suggestions are frequently accepted by children when explanations are provided and children are made to feel like they are a part of the decision making process.

There are many interventions parents can take toward pattern setting that are specific to infants and young children. It may seem unimportant while children are young, but these stages are actually vital. This is when patterns are initiated. Parents who teach their children to eat right and be active early on have healthier children who do not have to go through the struggle of changing patterns later in life.

Chapter 36

It's Not Too Late

This book largely focuses on prevention, but there are millions of children in this country who have already established unhealthy patterns. Changing negative patterns is more difficult than preventing them from occurring in the first place, but it definitely can be done.

Slow and Steady

Improving eating patterns takes time and cannot be rushed. When children and young adults undergo extreme dietary practices, growth and development may be sacrificed. Young people need fat for nerve development, protein for muscle and bone development, and carbohydrates to fuel bodies and brains. Strict diets may result in deficiencies that can lead to poor growth, weak bones, lack of energy, and difficulty learning. To effectively obtain and maintain ideal weight in a healthy fashion, positive eating patterns need to be established and maintained.

In order to improve eating and activity patterns, negative patterns must be replaced with positive ones. For a plan to be successful, transition is taken slowly. **The goal is "improvement over time."** When people have been raised with unhealthy patterns, the process of establishing healthy patterns will be frustrating. Drive, dedication, and a good support system are very helpful. One must remember weight gain is a process that occurs over time, and reversing the process takes time as well.

Motivation is the key factor for those who want to lose weight. Young people need to explore why this is important to them so they do not lose interest after a short period of time. Although a good support system is most helpful, young people must take personal responsibility for their dietary habits and exercise programs. Young people who are forced to diet by others will not be successful. The decision and drive to lose weight must come from within.

Reality of Success

Realistic goals and expectations should be set so older children who are overweight do not expect miracles and become disappointed by the slow process of weight loss. They need to be advised that weight should come off very slowly. A pound a week is an acceptable goal. Young adults may need reminding of the hazards of not eating enough healthy foods and of losing too much weight too fast. Unrealistic expectations set young people up for failure and sabotage the plan from the very beginning.

Behavior and habit modification is a must when attempting to lose weight. Recognizing and responding to the body's internal cues are very important. Unfortunately many people ignore such cues—they eat when they are not hungry and continue eating after becoming full. Eliminating such practices will amount to fewer consumed calories.

Stomach–Brain Connection

Eating slowly helps people recognize body cues. Correspondence between the stomach and brain can be rather slow. It takes 10 to 15 minutes from the time the stomach becomes full before the body recognizes it has enough food. During this processing time, fast eaters put away a lot more food than slower eaters do. People who eat slowly also enjoy food longer without taking in any more calories.

Minimizing distractions during eating is helpful in recognizing cues when they occur. When the mind is focused elsewhere, cues are often ignored and over-eating occurs. The outcome of recognizing and responding to internal cues may include weight loss, decreased stomach discomfort, and feelings of self-control.

Support for Success

Successful behavior and habit modification often depends on how family members interact with each other. Changing dietary patterns is tough, and everyone involved deserves positive reinforcement and praise.

Negative reinforcement should be avoided in all circumstances. Overweight young people should never be made to feel they are to blame for being over-weight. Instead, they can be told it is not their fault and reassured that something can be done about it. Kindness provides a huge emotional boost, especially for those having great difficulty making transitions.

Young people who are overweight frequently have a diminished self-esteem. It is vital parents treat self-esteem issues with care. Young people who are already disappointed in themselves do not need further ridicule from anyone, especially family members. Parents want what is best for their children and do not mean harm, but may make matters worse if they are overly concerned about their child's weight.

Although parents and family members must try their best not to say harmful things, there are times when constructive criticism may be necessary. At these times, it may be helpful to offer praise or positive comments as well. The feelings of young people who are attempting to lose weight can be hurt very easily. Family members can help them out by offering support, acceptance, and a lot of positive reinforcement.

Occupying Time

Spare time fosters snacking for many people. Social activities prevent this by keeping minds off food. Social activities can also improve one's outlook on life and improve self-esteem. Parents can help by taking part in social activities with their children. It is very helpful to find activities young people enjoy and can excel in. Sports or exercise-related activities are a great option as long as they are done with a nonjudgmental, supportive group. More mature young people may feel less intimidated and enjoy structured exercise classes for adults over those with peers.

Go for It

Eating properly and exercising is the most effective way to lose or maintain weight. Aerobic exercise is a must. It includes any exercise that uses the major muscles of the body nonstop for at least twenty minutes, not including the warm up and cool-down. This burns many calories and offers cardiovascular benefits. Once an aerobic routine is mastered, some individuals may choose to add resistance training for strength and body tone.

Resistance training, also called weightlifting, increases muscle mass. Since muscle burns more calories than fat does, individuals with a higher percentage of muscle constantly burn more calories than those with less muscle do. An increased muscle mass is a definite advantage for people who want to burn more calories.

Some parents shy away from starting their older children in weightlifting because they think their children, especially daughters, will develop large, unattractive muscles as seen on professional bodybuilders—this will not happen. In order to develop large muscles, most individuals would have to work out several hours every day. Even then most females will get somewhat larger and more defined muscles, but nowhere near what parents feel is too large or unattractive. It is helpful to know that most individuals who drastically increase muscle mass do so in an unnatural, unhealthy way—often with steroids and other enhancing drugs.

For most overweight children and young adults, maintaining an active lifestyle, as well as making proper food and beverage choices, is all that is needed to take excess weight off and keep it off. In extreme cases, young people may need specialized diets in addition to positive lifestyle changes. Such diets must be recommended and supervised by a physician.

Chapter 37

Get Ready, Get Set, Go

Each person and every family situation is unique; however, we all still have many things in common. Most parents will agree that among the commonalities we share are hopes for excellent health, happiness, and long life spans for our children and ourselves. In fact, most parents would do just about anything to be able to guarantee such gifts.

More commonalities parents frequently share are high stress, lack of time, and lack of energy. These constraints often prevent parents from accomplishing tasks that would make them and their children as healthy as possible. Although most parents have good intentions of doing what is best, reality can interfere.

Learning new skills takes time and effort, and establishing healthy patterns is no different. Fortunately with pattern setting, much of the time and effort required is only necessary during beginning stages. When healthy patterns are set, they usually do not require much more energy or effort to maintain than unhealthy patterns do. In fact, eating healthy foods and exercising regularly actually helps individuals cope with stress and increases energy levels.

Making health a priority and living life accordingly can be mastered in just a short amount of time, for those willing to initially put forth a little effort. The only requirements necessary to accomplish such goals are to retain the principles described in this book and commit to initiating and sticking with healthy patterns. Reaching and maintaining goals are always possible since parents choose the patterns and initiate them on their own time line. Although it is often impossible to drastically slow the pace of life, it is possible to use time more wisely, dedicating efforts toward obtaining and maintaining healthy patterns.

Success does not happen solely by reading or thinking about exercising and eating healthy foods—it requires action. First, parents need to get ready. This means deciding which goals can realistically be started now and how this will be accomplished. It is helpful to put such plans in writing. This solidifies the plan, helps parents remain accountable, and gives them something to refer back to from time to time.

Secondly, parents need to get set. This means using up or throwing away unhealthy foods in the home and replacing them with healthy foods. It also includes choosing which activities and exercise programs will be incorporated into daily life and when and where they will take place. Writing exercise dates on a calendar and having clothing and supplies gathered may be helpful.

When all of the preparation has been completed, it is time to get going. Congratulations on pursuing excellent family health and good luck on the journey there!

Label Language

Appendix A

Label Language

Many parents feel they do not have time to shop for and prepare fresh foods for their families, so they serve less healthy foods because they are quick and easy. By not making nutrition a priority, parents are trading convenience for the health of their families. Even when parents try to serve nutritious foods, it is often a struggle to figure out which are adequate choices. Processing and preparation can drastically change foods, so even when foods appear or are assumed to be healthy, they may not be. The ability to understand packaging labels is essential in choosing healthy foods over unhealthy foods.

Reading between the lines

Reading labels can be very confusing because consumers and food processors have different purposes for labels. Health-conscious consumers rely on food labels to inform them about products, and food processors use them to promote sales. Some food processors use conflicting interests to their advantage by using special captions on labels meant to draw attention to their products.

Unfortunately, many consumers are unaware that trendy wording frequently makes food sound much more healthy than it really is. Health-conscious people who are unfamiliar with reading labels are frequently fooled into purchasing foods that are not healthy choices. To avoid confusion, consumers must learn to understand how labeling works and examine fine print.

Translating the terminology

The first step in label reading is to ignore the front of the packaging. This area is designed for advertising, or in other words, to sell products. Here the truth can be stretched to make products sound like they are better for the body than they really are. Laws regulate the meanings of many terms, but manufacturers construe them to promote sales. Even though it is unlawful to lie on food labels, manufacturers can get away with stretching the truth. Being able to recognize such terms will prevent many consumers from being misled. Here is a list of some of the most frequently seen, misunderstood terms and their meanings:

- **And/or** means the product may contain one or all of the ingredients listed. Manufacturers may switch between ingredients several times during the year as price fluctuations occur. Often the least-healthy ingredients are the least-expensive ingredients, so they may be used more frequently. And/or labeling allows manufacturers to make switches between ingredients without changing what labels read.

- **Enriched** means synthetic nutrients are added, frequently after natural nutrients have been lost during processing.

- **Drink** or **cocktail** on fruit juice products usually means they contain little or no real fruit juice. They are often made of water, sugar, flavoring, and coloring. When purchasing juice, the label should always read "100% juice."

- **Concentrated** means the water has been removed. Usually the consumer puts water back in before use.

- **Energy** refers to any food or beverage that contains calories.

- **Free** means the food or beverage is absent of or contains a very small amount of something such as chemicals, cholesterol, calories, fat, sodium, or sugar.

- **Fresh** means uncooked, unprocessed, and frequently unfrozen.

- **Made from** means products start out as a particular food or foods. It does not mean those foods still contain their original nutrients. Many healthy foods are drastically changed during processing so the end product is less healthy, or even unhealthy.

- **Made with** means a particular ingredient was added. This is very misleading in that the amount added can be extremely small.

- **Natural** means nothing. Just about everything came from nature at one point or another, but it does not mean foods have not been processed or changed to a less healthy or unhealthy form.

- **Natural flavors** refers to flavors derived from nonsynthetic sources. They are used for taste rather than nutrition.

- **Pure** means nothing. Pure has no real meaning in food labeling and tells consumers absolutely nothing about a product.

Legally, virtually all food labels must provide consumers with the nutritional content of food. This benefits consumers who are conscientious about eating healthy foods, as well as those on special diets or that have food sensitivities. Parents who do not read labels or do not understand them have no idea what they are serving their families.

Once the skill of label reading is mastered, parents are often unpleasantly surprised at the amount of unhealthy foods their families consume on a regular basis. It is greatly to the consumer's benefit that laws require manufacturers to label products, but it is up to the consumer to make use of the information provided.

Nutrition facts

Unlike the front of packaging, the side and back of packaging contain factual information. In one of these spots, each product package contains a box that lists all of the nutrition facts. The law regulates what information is provided here, as well as how it is presented. This guarantees that information is provided, accurate, and easily compared to similar products.

All manufacturers must follow the same listing format—this allows the nutritional values of items to be compared with less difficulty. Consumers looking for nutritional information on any product should look at the "Nutrition Facts" panel first and compare with similar items when applicable.

Understanding labels —line by line

♦ Right under the Nutrition Facts heading is the **Serving Size** line. This line advises consumers of the amount of that particular product considered to be a single serving. Amounts listed are written in both common household units as well as metric measures. The serving size also tells consumers the amount of food to which all the other numbers on the Nutrition Facts panel apply. The Food and Drug Administration (FDA) sets guidelines for serving sizes so similar products will have similar serving sizes. Having uniform serving sizes makes comparing nutritional values less difficult. When comparing nutritional facts using the stated serving size, it is important for parents to remember that individuals of different ages, sizes, metabolisms, and activity levels eat different amounts. The serving size on labels may not be the amount each family member eats; therefore, appropriate calculations can be made to adjust nutritional facts according to the actual amount eaten.

♦ Next is the **Servings Per Container** line. It tells how many servings are in one container or package. This information enables consumers to figure out the cost per serving, and approximately how many people can be served from each package.

♦ The **Calorie** line tells how many calories are in one serving.

♦ The **Calories from Fat** line tells how many calories in one serving come from fat. Foods that get a large percentage of their calories from fat should be avoided or eaten in moderation.

♦ The block of text under the serving information is where the **Amount Per Serving (amount/serving)** column is found. This lists the amounts of calories, fats, cholesterol, sodium, carbohydrates, and protein in each serving. Other nutrients such as potassium may be added as well. Consumers can analyze these nutritional values to decide if the values

(Exhibit 1) **Sample Label**

WHOLE-WHEAT BREAD

Nutrition Facts

Serving Size: 1 Slice (40g)

Servings Per Container: 17

Calories 120

Calories from Fat: 10

Amount/serving	%Daily Value*
Total Fat 1g	1%
Saturated Fat 0g	0%
Cholesterol 0mg	0%
Sodium 190mg	8%
Total Carbohydrate 18g	6%
Dietary Fiber 3g	11%
Sugars 2g	
Protein 4g	
Vitamin A	0%
Vitamin C	0%
Calcium	4%
Iron	4%
Thiamin	8%
Riboflavin	8%
Niacin	15%
Folate	0%

*Percent Daily Values are based on a 2,000 calorie diet. Your daily values may be higher or lower depending on your calorie needs.

	Calories	2,000	2,500
Total Fat	Less than	65g	80g
Sat Fat	Less than	20g	25g
Cholesterol	Less than	300mg	300mg
Sodium	Less than	2,400mg	2,400mg
Potassium	Less than	3,500mg	3,500mg
Total Carbohydrate		300g	375g
Dietary Fiber		25g	30g
Protein		50g	65g

Calories per Gram:

Fat 9 • Carbohydrate 4 • Protein 4

INGREDIENTS: WHOLE WHEAT FLOUR, WATER, HIGH FRUCTOSE CORN SYRUP, WHEAT GLUTEN, YEAST, CRUSHED WHEAT, CONTAINS 2% OR LESS OF THE FOLLOWING: CANOLA AND/OR SOYBEAN OIL, MOLASSES, WHEAT BRAN, SALT, WHEY, CALCIUM SULFATE, DOUGH CONDITIONERS (MAY CONTAIN ONE OR MORE OF THE FOLLOWING: SODIUM STEAROYL LACTYLATE, DATEM, SOY FLOUR), MONO- AND DIGLYCERIDES.

meet personal dietary requirements for individuals and families. The information provided is very useful for comparing similar items when shopping for healthy foods. Such comparisons are often very simple when serving sizes listed are identical. When serving sizes listed differ from serving sizes consumed, the values in this listing will be decreased or increased accordingly.

♦ The **Total Fat** line tells how many grams of fat are in one serving.

♦ The **Saturated Fat** line (a subheading under Total Fat) tells how many grams of saturated fat are in one serving.

♦ The **Cholesterol** line tells how many milligrams of cholesterol are in one serving. This line leaves out some important information for those who monitor their cholesterol. It does not include the amounts of cholesterol-raising fats. Individuals concerned about cholesterol can look for fats to avoid, such as partially hydrogenated oils, in the ingredient listing. Foods with large or moderate amounts of cholesterol and cholesterol-raising fats should be avoided or eaten in moderation.

♦ The **Sodium** line tells how many milligrams of sodium are in one serving.

♦ The **Potassium** line tells how many milligrams of potassium are in one serving. This line may or may not appear on food labels. It is a voluntary listing and not legally required.

♦ The **Total Carbohydrate** line tells how many grams of total carbohydrates are in one serving. Carbohydrates are further broken down by subheadings that follow. This allows consumers to differentiate good and bad carbohydrates.

♦ The **Dietary Fiber** line (a subheading under Total Carbohydrate) tells how many grams of fiber are in one serving.

♦ The **Sugars** line (another subheading under Total Carbohydrate) tells how many grams of sugars are in one serving. Sugars include those naturally present in foods such as lactose in milk and fructose in fruits, as well as those added to food such as table sugar, corn syrup, and dextrose. Consumers can compare this line to the Total Carbohydrate line on the food label to determine how much of the carbohydrates in a particular food are from naturally present sugars or added sugars. When the numbers listed on the Total Carbohydrate line and the Sugars line are the same or fairly close together, much of the carbohydrates are from added sugars. Such products tend to be junk foods and should be avoided or eaten in moderation. There are a few exceptions to this rule. They occur with foods like milk, fruit, and 100% fruit juice. These products contain natural sugars. Like junk food labels, these will have little or no discrepancy between the Total Carbohydrate and Sugars lines. In contrast, when there is a high Total Carbohydrate amount and a low sugar amount, consumers can assume the food contains mostly complex carbohydrates and little or no added sugar. Comparing the carbohydrate values is beneficial for health-conscious consumers.

♦ The **Other Carbohydrate** line (another subheading under Total Carbohydrate) tells how many grams of carbohydrates, other than those listed under the Dietary Fiber and Sugars subheadings, a serving of a particular product contains. This heading includes complex carbohydrates (excluding fiber) and other sugars that are naturally present in foods. This line may not appear on some labels.

♦ The **Protein** line tells how many grams of protein are in one serving.

♦ The next block of text is the **Vitamins and Minerals** area. It provides percentages of recommended daily values of vitamins A and C, iron, and calcium a serving of a particular product contains. Other vitamins and minerals may be listed as well but are not legally required.

♦ To the right of "Amount Per Serving" is a separate listing titled **% Daily Value.** This lists percentages of the daily requirements of each nutritional value (Total Fat, Saturated Fat, Cholesterol, Sodium, Total Carbohydrate, and Dietary Fiber) one serving of the food provides. The percentage of recommended daily value for protein is not listed because protein insufficiency is not a concern to most individuals. The daily values listed are based on a daily 2,000-calorie diet and are intended for individuals over four years of age. Individuals who consume more or less than 2,000 calories a day can adjust percentages accordingly.

Understanding how ingredients are listed

A list of ingredients contained in a product is printed near the manufacturer's label on the side or back of that product's packaging—this is required by the Food and Drug Administration. Such ingredients must be listed in descending order of predominance. In other words, each individual package must display its ingredients in order from those that weigh the most to those that weigh the least. The list is very important in determining what ingredients and how much of each the product contains.

The ingredient listing is a source of information especially useful for health-conscious people, and for those with food sensitivities. Health-conscious individuals can use the descending order of predominance rule to determine if unhealthy ingredients, like saturated fats, are contained in small amounts or in excessive amounts—this can clearly help consumers choose which foods they will, and will not, purchase.

Some manufacturers list more than one ingredient using labels such as **and/or** and **contains one or more of the following**. This type of labeling does not inform consumers of actual product ingredients, and can create problems for health-conscious consumers.

For example: Two different oils may be listed on a product with **and/or** labeling. One oil may be healthy and one may be harmful. Unfortunately, consumers do not know which oil or oils are actually in the product.

Only under certain conditions does the FDA permit using nonspecific labeling. The manufacturers must be unable to predict which of the listed ingredients will be used, and the quantities used must be very small. Such labels are tricky and do not benefit consumers—some individuals choose to avoid purchasing products with labels that are nonspecific.

Ingredient lists of some products will contain unfamiliar terms. Many of these ingredients are fats, sweeteners, preservatives, additives, flavors, and colorings—some artificial, some not. With so many different scientific terms, it is difficult for the consumer to consistently determine which are healthy and which are not. Luckily, ingredients of this type are usually at the very end of the ingredient list, so it can be assumed that only very small amounts are present, although this is not always the case. Products containing numerous unknown terms may be better left in the marketplace. When in doubt, it is best to choose products that are closest to their natural state.

Health and nutrition claims

Health and nutrition claims are new food labels that describe how certain nutrients or foods can negatively or positively affect disease or health-related conditions. Approved claims that can be used on labels include:

♦ calcium and a lower risk of osteoporosis

♦ fat and a greater risk of cancer

♦ saturated fat and cholesterol and a greater risk of coronary heart disease

♦ fiber containing grain products, fruits, and vegetables and a reduced risk of cancer

♦ fruits, vegetables, and grain products containing fiber and a reduced risk of coronary heart disease

♦ sodium and a greater risk of high blood pressure

♦ fruits and vegetables and a reduced risk of cancer

♦ folic acid and a decreased risk of neural tube defect-affected pregnancy

Health and Nutrient Claims are truthful and can only be used under certain circumstances, such as when a particular food contains appropriate amounts of stated nutrients.

Comparing labels

Comparing labels is the best way to decipher the nutritional difference between packaged products. When comparing values and ingredients, consumers can quickly determine which products to leave at the marketplace and which to take home.

Cereal label comparison

Cereal can be one of the healthiest foods eaten—or pure junk. Some types are obviously one or the other, but many fall somewhere in between. To determine if particular cereals are nutritionally worth purchasing, their labels must be read and compared to others (see exhibit 2).

Here are some general facts on the example cereal panels to make note of:

◆ There is a difference in serving size—the nutritious cereal has a 1-cup (49 grams) serving size; the junk cereal has a ¾-cup (26 grams) serving size. If the boxes of cereals were close in nutritional value, the serving size would have to be considered in the comparison of nutritional value. Since the first box of cereal is obviously more nutritious, close evaluation is not needed.

◆ On the cereal panels, a separate list of nutritional percentages are offered for values of the cereal with added fat-free milk.

◆ The healthy cereal has slightly more calories than the junk food cereal. This is because one serving of the healthy cereal is larger and heavier. Nutritional choices cannot be made based solely on the amount of calories that foods contain.

> **For example:** When compared to sugary cereals, a higher calorie nutritious cereal may take less to create the sensation of fullness, more time to digest, and keep energy levels stable for longer periods of time.

◆ The healthy cereal contains no sodium—the junk cereal contains 105 mg.

◆ The healthy cereal contains 200 mg of potassium—the junk cereal contains 50 mg.

◆ The healthy cereal contains 40 grams of total carbohydrates—the junk cereal contains 23 grams. This information alone does not inform the consumer if carbohydrates are healthy (like whole grains) or unhealthy (like excessive sugars). To figure out which is better, consumers can look directly under the carbohydrate line. The healthy cereal contains fibers and other carbohydrates with absolutely no added sugar. This means the 40 grams of carbohydrates are all from sources that greatly benefit the body. In contrast, the junk cereal contains 11 grams of sugar out of only 23 grams of total carbohydrates—this tells consumers sugar is a main ingredient in the junk cereal. The ingredient listing confirms this—sugar is the first ingredient listed, which means there is more sugar than any other ingredient.

◆ The healthy cereal contains 6 grams of protein—the junk cereal contains only 1 gram.

(Exhibit 2) Cereal Label Comparison: Nutritious vs. Unhealthy

NUTRITIOUS CEREAL

Nutrition Facts

Serving Size: 1 cup (49g)
Servings Per Container: about 10

Amount per serving	Cereal	Cereal with ½ cup Fat-free Milk
Calories	170	210
Calories from Fat:	10	10
	%Daily Value**	
Total Fat 1g*	2%	2%
Saturated Fat 0g	0%	0%
Polyunsaturated Fat 0.5g		
Monounsaturated Fat 0g		
Cholesterol 0mg	0%	0%
Sodium 0mg	0%	3%
Potassium 200mg	6%	11%
Total Carbohydrate 40g	13%	15%
Dietary Fiber 6g	24%	24%
Soluble Fiber 1g		
Insoluble Fiber 5g		
Sugars 0g		
Other Carbohydrates 34g		
Protein 6g		
Vitamin A	0%	4%
Vitamin C	0%	2%
Calcium	2%	15%
Iron	8%	8%
Thiamin	10%	15%
Riboflavin	2%	10%
Niacin	5%	15%
Vitamin B6	4%	6%
Folic Acid	4%	4%
Phosphorus	20%	30%
Magnesium	15%	20%
Zinc	10%	15%
Copper	8%	8%

*Amount in cereal. ½ cup fat-free milk contributes an additional 40 calories, 65mg sodium, 200mg potassium, 6g total carbohydrates (6g sugars), and 4g protein.

**Percent Daily Values are based on a 2,000 calorie diet. Your daily values may be higher or lower depending on your calorie needs.

	Calories	2,000	2,500
Total Fat	Less than	65g	80g
Sat Fat	Less than	20g	25g
Cholesterol	Less than	300mg	300mg
Sodium	Less than	2,400mg	2,400mg
Potassium	Less than	3,500mg	3,500mg
Total Carbohydrate		300g	375g
Dietary Fiber		25g	30g

INGREDIENTS: WHOLE-GRAIN WHEAT. TO PRESERVE THE NATURAL WHEAT FLAVOR, BHT IS ADDED TO THE PACKAGING MATERIAL.

UNHEALTHY CEREAL

Nutrition Facts

Serving Size: ¾ cup (26g)
Servings Per Container: about 14

Amount per serving	Cereal	Cereal with ½ cup Fat-free Milk
Calories	100	140
Calories from Fat:	10	10
	%Daily Value**	
Total Fat 1g*	2%	2%
Saturated Fat 0g	0%	0%
Cholesterol 0mg	0%	0%
Sodium 105mg	4%	7%
Potassium 50mg	1%	7%
Total Carbohydrate 23g	8%	10%
Dietary Fiber 1g	3%	3%
Sugars 11g		
Other Carbohydrates 11g		
Protein 1g		
Vitamin A	10%	15%
Vitamin C	10%	10%
Calcium	0%	15%
Iron	25%	25%
Thiamin	25%	25%
Riboflavin	25%	35%
Niacin	25%	25%
Vitamin B6	25%	25%
Folic Acid	100%	100%
Zinc	25%	30%

*Amount in cereal. ½ cup fat-free milk contributes an additional 40 calories, 65mg sodium, 200mg potassium, 6g total carbohydrates (6g sugars), and 4g protein.

**Percent Daily Values are based on a 2,000 calorie diet. Your daily values may be higher or lower depending on your calorie needs.

	Calories	2,000	2,500
Total Fat	Less than	65g	80g
Sat Fat	Less than	20g	25g
Cholesterol	Less than	300mg	300mg
Sodium	Less than	2,400mg	2,400mg
Potassium	Less than	3,500mg	3,500mg
Total Carbohydrate		300g	375g
Dietary Fiber		25g	30g

INGREDIENTS: SUGAR, CORN FLOUR, WHOLE OAT FLOUR, CORN SYRUP SOLIDS, PARTIALLY HYDRO-GENATED COTTON-SEED OIL, CORN STARCH, COCOA (PROCESSED WITH ALKALI), SALT, CARAMEL COLOR, NATURAL AND ARTIFICIAL FLAVORS, CONFEC-TIONER'S GLAZE, YELLOW 6, SODIUM ASCORBATE (A VITAMIN C SOURCE), RED 40, NIACINAMIDE*, REDUCED IRON, ZINC OXIDE, YELLOW 5, RED 3, BLUE1, VITAMIN A PALMITATE, CARNAUBA WAX, BLUE 2, GREEN 3, THIAMIN MONONITRATE*, PYRIDOXINE HYDROCHLORIDE*, BHT (A PRESERVATIVE), RIBO-FLAVIN*, FOLIC ACID, **ONE OF THE B VITAMINS.

♦ When comparing the vitamin and mineral listing between the two cereals, consumers may be very disillusioned—the junk cereal appears to have significantly more vitamins and minerals than the healthy cereal does. How can this be when the healthy cereal is made with far superior ingredients? The answer can be found in the ingredient listing of the junk cereal. Since the cereal itself contains very few nutrients, synthetic vitamins and minerals are added. Some consumers purchase products by analyzing only the vitamin and mineral category. What they do not realize is that products in a more natural state are often more slowly, more completely, and more thoroughly utilized by the body than foods in unnatural states. In addition some of the vitamins added to foods such as sugary cereals are poorly absorbed by the body and never reach the bloodstream at all.

♦ Ingredient comparison needs little explanation. The healthy cereal contains whole-grain wheat, and special packaging is used to maintain the natural wheat flavor—period, that's it. The junk cereal, on the other hand, contains mostly sugar, flour (corn and whole oat), corn syrup solids (more sugar), and partially hydrogenated cottonseed oil (trans fat—harmful to the body). The other two-thirds of the ingredients are flavorings, colorings, preservatives, and vitamin additives— none of which does the body much good. This product and many other junk foods contain artificial colorings that can be identified by an actual color name with a number after it. Examples of these are yellow 6, red 40, red 3, and blue 1. Such colorings are generally recognized as safe, but complete safety has not yet been established. Parents who have children with food sensitivities or behavior problems may choose to limit products that contain artificial substances.

Juice label comparison

The front of juice containers can be quite deceptive, so consumers need to read labels to determine which juices are nutritious and which are not. As with the cereal example, those who read labels can easily determine which is which.

Here are some general facts on the juice labels (exhibit 3) to make note of:

♦ The serving size of these examples must be read in milliliters since one choice comes as small individual-serving-sized pouches and the other is measured as 8-ounce servings. In this case, serving sizes are similar. Some manufacturers list smaller amounts as serving sizes because they can then list lesser amounts of the values consumers frequently compare, such as calories, fat, sodium, and carbohydrates. Consumers with limited label-reading skills may mistake lower-calorie choices as preferable products.

♦ Calories of the 100% orange juice are 110 per serving—calories of the juice drink are 100. This is about equal considering the difference in serving-size, but if unsure, the milliliter per serving can be divided by the calories per serving to obtain the calories per milliliter. These amounts can then be compared to each other.

(Exhibit 3) Juice Label Comparison:
100% Pure Orange Juice vs. Orange Juice Drink

100% ORANGE JUICE	
Pure Orange Juice	
Contains 100% Orange Juice	
Nutrition Facts	
Serving Size: 8 fl. oz (240mL)	
Servings Per Container: 8	
Calories: 110 per serving	
Calories from Fat 0	
Amount per serving	%Daily Value*
Total Fat 0g	0%
Sodium 0mg	0%
Potassium 450 mg	13%
Total Carbohydrate 26g	9%
Sugars 22g	
Protein 2g	
Vitamin C	120%
Calcium	2%
Thiamin	10%
Riboflavin	4%
Niacin	6%
Vitamin B6	6%
Folate	15%
Magnesium	6%

*Percent Daily Values are based on a 2,000 calorie diet.

Naturally sodium free.

No water or preservatives added.

INGREDIENTS: 100% PURE ORANGE JUICE.

While many factors affect heart disease, a diet that is low in total fat, saturated fat and cholesterol combined with a healthy lifestyle may reduce the risk of heart disease.

Diets containing foods that are good sources of potassium and low in sodium may reduce the risk of high blood pressure and stroke.

ORANGE DRINK	
All Natural Juice Drink	
Contains 10% Fruit Juice	
Nutrition Facts	
Serving Size: 1 pouch (200mL)	
Servings Per Container: 10	
Calories: 100 per serving	
Amount per serving	%Daily Value*
Total Fat 0g	0%
Sodium 20mg	1%
Total Carbohydrate 25g	1%
Sugars 25g	
Protein 0g	

*Percent Daily Values are based on a 2,000 calorie diet.

INGREDIENTS: WATER, HIGH FRUCTOSE CORN SYRUP, WATER EXTRACTED ORANGE JUICE CONCENTRATE, CITRIC ACID, NATURAL FLAVOR.

- Sodium is 0 in the 100% juice—it is 20 mg per serving in the juice drink.

- Potassium is 450 mg in the 100% juice—it is not listed on the juice drink panel. This probably means there is very little to no potassium in the juice drink.(Potassium listing is optional on labels.)

- Total carbohydrates are 26 grams with 22 grams of sugar in the 100% juice—carbohydrates are 25 grams with 25 grams of sugar in the juice drink. Since the number of grams of sugar and carbohydrates in each product is high, we know there is a lot of sugar in both beverages. The 100% juice is all juice, so the 22 grams of sugar are natural sugars and the 4 grams that are not are obviously other natural, healthy components of the fruit. Although this 100% juice is very nutritious, it does contain a lot of natural sugars that are caloric. Even great sources of nutrition such as these should be limited to reduce sugar and calories consumed (diluting is advised). On the contrary, since the juice drink contains equal amounts of total carbohydrates and sugar, and we can see by the ingredient listing that the carbohydrates are not from fruit sources, consumers know all or most of the carbohydrates in the product come from added sugar. Obviously, this drink is mostly flavored sugar water—this fact can be confirmed by looking at the ingredient label.

- Protein in the 100% juice is 2 grams—there is none in the juice drink.

- Vitamins and minerals are in abundance in the 100% juice— the juice drink lists absolutely none.

- Ingredients between the two beverages differ like night and day. The 100% juice contains nothing but juice—no water or preservatives have been added. In contrast, the fruit drink consists of water, high fructose corn syrup (sugar), citric acid, and flavorings that may or may not be natural.

- Unlike that of the juice drink, the packaging of the 100% juice product offers two "Nutrient Claims." They are: "Diets containing foods that are good sources of potassium and low in sodium may reduce the risk of high blood pressure and stroke" and "While many factors affect heart disease, a diet that is low in total fat, saturated fat, and cholesterol combined with a healthy lifestyle may reduce the risk of heart disease." Nutrient Claims are a big bonus.

Whole-wheat, wheat, and white bread label comparison

Many people think wheat bread and whole-wheat bread are one and the same. By comparing labels, it becomes obvious whole-wheat bread is much more nutritious than wheat, and wheat bread is almost identical to white.

The nutritional differences between breads are not easily detected by examining the nutritional values on labels. This is because synthetic nutrients are added to white flour in order to replace some of the nutrients lost during processing and bleaching. Synthetic vitamins and minerals do not replace all the natural goodness of whole-wheat flour.

By looking at the first line or two on any ingredient listing, consumers can differentiate between healthy and unhealthy breads. The type of flour is what makes the difference.

Here are some general facts on bread labels (exhibit 4) to make note of:

♦ Since the white and wheat breads are made with enriched flour, the nutrients listed in their labels' Nutritional Facts columns look similar to those on the whole-wheat label. The quickest way to choose bread is to look for the heading *100% whole-wheat* or *100% whole-grain* on the front of the package. Consumers who desire more verification or information can read the ingredient listings.

♦ The ingredients listed for the white and wheat breads are very similar. On both, the first ingredient is enriched flour, followed by a breakdown of added synthetic nutrients. (This is where the vitamins in the Nutrition Facts come from.) In contrast, the first ingredient in the 100% whole-wheat bread is whole-wheat flour, which has not lost its original nutrients through processing. Basically, consumers can make healthy bread choices by understanding this alone.

♦ Many people believe wheat bread is just a shortened way of saying whole-wheat bread—this is not so. Wheat bread is actually very close to white bread. When comparing labels of wheat and white breads, consumers can see the only difference between the two is that a touch of whole-wheat flour, wheat bran (not 100%), and molasses (probably for color) was added to white enriched flour. Such findings will show consumers most wheat breads offer little or no benefit over white bread.

♦ The whole-wheat bread has 120 calories and the other two have 70. This is not a negative point (even for calorie counters), because the whole-wheat bread is 40 grams per serving and the wheat and white breads are only 29 grams per serving. One serving of the whole-wheat bread would be much more filling and keep the stomach full longer. This could actually result in fewer daily calories consumed.

(Exhibit 4) Bread Label Comparison: Whole-Wheat vs. Wheat vs. White

WHOLE-WHEAT

Nutrition Facts

Serving Size: 1 Slice (40g)

Servings Per Container: 17

Calories 120

Calories from Fat: 10

Amount/serving	%Daily Value*
Total Fat 1g	1%
Saturated Fat 0g	0%
Cholesterol 0mg	0%
Sodium 190mg	8%
Total Carbohydrate 18g	6%
Dietary Fiber 3g	11%
Sugars 2g	
Protein 4g	
Vitamin A	0%
Vitamin C	0%
Calcium	4%
Iron	4%
Thiamin	8%
Riboflavin	8%
Niacin	15%
Folate	0%

*Percent Daily Values are based on a 2,000 calorie diet. Your daily values may be higher or lower depending on your calorie needs.

	Calories	2,000	2,500
Total Fat	Less than	65g	80g
Sat Fat	Less than	20g	25g
Cholesterol	Less than	300mg	300mg
Sodium	Less than	2,400mg	2,400mg
Potassium	Less than	3,500mg	3,500mg
Total Carbohydrate		300g	375g
Dietary Fiber		25g	30g
Protein		50g	65g

Calories per Gram:

Fat 9 • Carbohydrate 4 • Protein 4

INGREDIENTS: WHOLE WHEAT FLOUR, WATER, HIGH FRUCTOSE CORN SYRUP, WHEAT GLUTEN, YEAST, CRUSHED WHEAT, CONTAINS 2% OR LESS OF THE FOLLOWING: CANOLA AND/OR SOYBEAN OIL, MOLASSES, WHEAT BRAN, SALT, WHEY, CALCIUM SULFATE, DOUGH CONDITIONERS (MAY CONTAIN ONE OR MORE OF THE FOLLOWING: SODIUM STEAROYL LACTYLATE, DATEM, SOY FLOUR), MONO- AND DIGLYCERIDES.

WHEAT

Nutrition Facts

Serving Size: 1 Slice (29g)

Servings Per Container: 22

Calories 70

Calories from Fat: 5

Amount/serving	%Daily Value*
Total Fat 1g	1%
Saturated Fat 0g	0%
Cholesterol 0mg	0%
Sodium 150mg	6%
Total Carborhydrate 13g	5%
Dietary Fiber 1g	2%
Sugars 1g	
Protein 2g	
Vitamin A	0%
VitaminC	0%
Calcium	0%
Iron	4%
Thiamin	8%
Riboflavin	4%
Niacin	6%
Folate	6%

*Percent Daily Values are based on a 2,000 calorie diet. Your daily values may be higher or lower depending on your calorie needs.

	Calories	2,000	2,500
Total Fat	Less than	65g	80g
Sat Fat	Less than	20g	25g
Cholesterol	Less than	300mg	300mg
Sodium	Less than	2,400mg	2,400mg
Potassium	Less than	3,500mg	3,500mg
Total Carbohydrate		300g	375g
Dietary Fiber		25g	30g
Protein		50g	65g

Calories per Gram:

Fat 9 • Carbohydrate 4 • Protein 4

INGREDIENTS: ENRICHED FLOUR (WHEAT FLOUR, MALTED BARLEY FLOUR, IRON, NIACIN, THIAMIN MONONITRATE, RIBOFLAVIN, FOLIC ACID), WATER, WHEAT BRAN, HIGH FRUCTOSE CORN SYRUP, WHOLE-WHEAT FLOUR, CONTAINS 2% OR LESS OF THE FOLLOWING: BUTTER, MOLASSES, WHEAT GLUTEN, YEAST, CANOLA AND/OR SOYBEAN OIL, SALT, CALCUIM SULFATE, NATURAL FLAVORS, CULTURED WHEY, DOUGH CONDITIONERS (MAY CONTAIN ONE OR MORE OF THE FOLLOWING: SODIUM STEAROYL LACTYLATE, ETHOXYLATED MONO- AND DIGLYCERIDES, MONOCALCIUM PHOSPHATE, DATEM, SOY FLOUR), MONO- AND DIGLYCERIDES, VINEGAR.

WHITE

Nutrition Facts

Serving Size: 1 Slice (29g)

Servings Per Container: 22

Calories 70

Calories from Fat: 5

Amount/serving	%Daily Value*
Total Fat 1g	1%
Saturated Fat 0g	0%
Cholesterol 0mg	0%
Sodium 140mg	6%
Total Carbohydrate 14g	5%
Dietary Fiber 1g	2%
Sugars 1g	
Protein 2g	
Vitamin A	0%
Vitamin C	0%
Calcium	2%
Iron	4%
Thiamin	8%
Riboflavin	4%
Niacin	4%
Folate	6%

*Percent Daily Values are based on a 2,000 calorie diet. Your daily values may be higher or lower depending on your calorie needs.

	Calories	2,000	2,500
Total Fat	Less than	65g	80g
Sat Fat	Less than	20g	25g
Cholesterol	Less than	300mg	300mg
Sodium	Less than	2,400mg	2,400mg
Potassium	Less than	3,500mg	3,500mg
Total Carbohydrate		300g	375g
Dietary Fiber		25g	30g
Protein		50g	65g

Calories per Gram:

Fat 9 • Carbohydrate 4 • Protein 4

INGREDIENTS: ENRICHED FLOUR (WHEAT FLOUR, MALTED BARLEY FLOUR, IRON, NIACIN, THIAMIN MONONITRATE, RIBOFLAVIN, FOLIC ACID), WATER, HIGH FRUCTOSE CORN SYRUP, CONTAINS 2% OR LESS OF EACH OF THE FOLLOWING: BUTTER, CANOLA AND/OR SOYBEAN OIL, YEAST, SALT, CALCIUM SULFATE, NATURAL FLAVORS, CULTURED WHEY, DOUGH CONDITIONERS (MAY CONTAIN ONE OR MORE OF THE FOLLOWING: SODIUM STEAROYL LACTYLATE, ETHOXYLATED MONO- AND DIGLYCERIDES, MONOCALCIUM PHOSPHATE, DATEM, SOY FLOUR), MONO- AND DIGLYCERIDES, VINEGAR.

♦ The "and/or rule" was described earlier. Each of the bread examples presented here lists canola oil and/or soybean oil in the ingredients. Individuals who wish to avoid such labeling can do so by reading various whole-wheat bread labels until they find a manufacturer who lists only the actual ingredients used. Those who are not overly bothered by the labeling technique can be reassured the amounts of the oils used are minimal.

Although 100% whole-wheat and 100% whole-grain are the healthiest breads, health-conscious consumers are not limited to eating the same bread all the time—there are many choices. Health-food shops and specialty shops often sell a variety of 100% whole-wheat breads and many are even healthier than commercial brands. They frequently contain the best oils and no artificial flavors, colors, additives, preservatives, or *and/or* labeling. The label below (exhibit 5) is one of many examples of such breads:

(Exhibit 5) **Sample Specialty Bread Label**

WHOLE-WHEAT BREAD
Contains: whole-wheat flour, water,
bran, pumpernickel, canola oil,
sea salt, yeast.
All natural, no preservatives.

Special labeling on food for children

As with cereal, juice, and bread, most other foods are intended for adults as well as children. However, there are foods designed and marketed just for children under the age of four. Regulations for children's foods state manufacturers must include nutritional information like amounts of fats, sodium, carbohydrates, protein, vitamins, and minerals on applicable labels. Such ingredient listings help parents choose appropriate types and amounts of foods most beneficial for their children.

(Exhibit 6) **Sample Baby-Food Label**

Nutrition Facts	Amount Per Serving		Amount Per Serving	
Serving Size	Total Fat	0g	Total Carb	10g
1 Jar (113g)	Sodium	55mg	Dietary Fiber	2g
Calories 45			Sugars	7g
			Protein	1g

%Daily Value: Protein 0%   Vitamin A 150%   Vitamin C 0%   Calcium 4%   Iron 0%

Ingredients: Organic Carrots, Water.

Label regulations on food for children under the age of four cannot show how the amounts of some nutrients correspond to Daily Values. This is because some nutrients such as fat, fiber, and sodium do not have Daily Values established for children under four. Daily Values for vitamins, minerals, and protein for this age group are established and displayed on packaging labels. Such regulations apply to most foods intended for infants and toddlers. Items include baby foods, infant beverages, teething biscuits, infant juices, and infant cereals. They do not include baby formula, which has its own special nutrition-labeling requirements.

There are many allowed facts on food labels for children under the age of four—and disallowed facts as well. Parents can be reassured most rules are made in the best interest of young children. A benefit to less information appearing on labels is they are easier to read. The baby-food label on the previous page (exhibit 6) is an example of how brief such labels can be.

Label summation

Learning to read labels is one of the larger steps parents can take to improve the dietary intake of their families. It takes time and effort, like learning anything else, but it is not difficult. To begin, parents can choose values most important to them and begin their focus there. As time goes by and parents become comfortable reading labels, the focus can be broadened to a more in-depth comparison of nutritional facts.

Grocery Guidance

Appendix B

Appendix B

Grocery Guidance

Before parents can serve healthy foods, they must know what to purchase. This sounds simple, but actually can be mind-boggling when faced with thousands of products on grocery-store shelves. The thought of reading labels might seem impossible for those who do not know where to start.

This "grocery list" of very healthy items has been prepared for parents who would like a little additional help. The list provides parents with a starting point. Each family can personalize and expand upon it as they wish.

Produce section
✔ Fresh fruits
✔ Fresh vegetables
✔ Tofu
✔ Soy hot dogs
✔ Fresh herbs and spices
✔ Vegetable juices
✔ Nuts

Dairy/Refrigerator section
✔ Low-fat organic milk
✔ Low-fat soy milk
✔ Low-fat yogurt
✔ Cheese
✔ Low-fat cottage cheese
✔ Low-fat cream cheese
✔ Eggs
✔ Egg substitute
✔ 100% orange juice, not from concentrate
✔ Corn tortillas

Beverage aisle
✔ 100% fruit juice
✔ Sports drinks

Canned food aisle

✔ Canned vegetables
✔ Canned fruit—in its own juice
✔ Canned beans
✔ Olives
✔ Canned tuna—packed in water
✔ Canned salmon
✔ Sardines
✔ Reduced-salt soups
✔ Low-salt broth

Cereal aisle

✔ Low-sugar, whole-grain cereal
✔ Unsweetened and unflavored oatmeal

Snack aisle

✔ Whole-wheat crackers
✔ Low-fat granola bars
✔ Nuts
✔ Popcorn kernels
✔ Whole-wheat bread sticks
✔ Dried fruit
✔ Applesauce—with no added sugar

Meat and Seafood section

✔ Fish
✔ Turkey
✔ Chicken
✔ Lean red meat

Bread aisle

(all whole-wheat or whole-grain)

✔ Bread
✔ Bagels
✔ English muffins
✔ Flour tortillas
✔ Pita bread

Packaged food aisle
- ✔ Whole- wheat pasta
- ✔ Brown rice
- ✔ Dried beans

Condiment aisle
- ✔ Natural peanut butter
- ✔ Low-fat salad dressing
- ✔ Fat-free mayonnaise
- ✔ Mustard
- ✔ Ketchup
- ✔ 100% fruit jam

Delicatessen section
- ✔ Rotisserie chicken
- ✔ Lean, unprocessed cold cuts
- ✔ Hummus
- ✔ Tofu pate

Cooking/Baking aisle
- ✔ Non-stick spray
- ✔ Virgin olive oil
- ✔ Low-salt spices
- ✔ Whole-wheat pancake and waffle mix

Frozen food section
- ✔ Frozen fish
- ✔ Frozen vegetables
- ✔ Frozen fruit
- ✔ 100% fruit-juice popsicles
- ✔ Low-fat frozen yogurt
- ✔ Low-fat ice cream

Pharmacy
- ✔ Toothbrushes with rotating head
- ✔ Children's toothpaste
- ✔ Dental floss
- ✔ Chewable multivitamins (if age-appropriate)

— DEDICATION —

To all of the parents who love their children
so much that they are willing to put forth
extra energy and commitment into making
them as happy and healthy as possible!

Index